Race Redomra

First edition published in Australia 2019
© Race Redomra 2019

Cover Design by Rocio Martin Osuna
Typeset by Rocio Martin Osuna
Back cover head shot by Isabelle Creative Media
Stock images used designed by Freepik and by Macrovector / Freepik

Paperback ISBN# 978-0-6485825-0-2
Ebook ISBN# 978-0-6485825-1-9

All persons interviewed including contributors to this book, have provided their content with consent. Resource websites are acknowledged and credited.
Any inaccuracies that may have occurred during the editing process, can be rectified in the 2nd addition with corrections and acknowledgments.

Disclaimer

The material in this publication is of the nature of general comment only, and does not represent professional advice. It is not intended to provide specific guidance for particular circumstances and it should not be relied on as the basis for any decision to take action or not take action on a matter which it covers. Readers should obtain professional advice where appropriate, before making any such decision. To the maximum extent permitted by law, the author and publisher disclaim all responsibility and liability to any person, arising directly or indirectly from any person taking or not taking action based on the information in this publication.

FIT AND CHILLED OUT

The author acknowledges the Traditional Custodians of the past, present and emerging on whose land this book was conceived, written and produced.

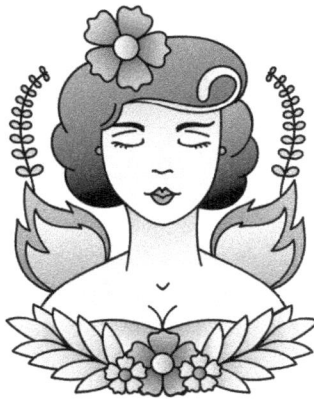

Bio

Describing herself as the 'pink sheep among the black sheep', and seldom feeling as though she wholly fit in anywhere, author Race Redomra can attest to the profound importance of self-discovery as a stepping-stone to authentic, meaningful living. Since her childhood, Race has known that she did not desire to swim comfortably down the stream of life, with the mainstream current carrying her on a safe, predictable journey.

Born a highly sensitive empath, Race noticed from an early age that she could sense the true feelings and intentions of the people around her. This trait gave Race a certain magnetism, and people have been drawn to her compassionate nature throughout her life. However, her ability to discern other peoples' truths wasn't always met with love and acceptance. As a result, Race has survived (and thrived in spite of) some profound challenges. The worlds of dance, martial arts, and meditation became safe spaces where Race could direct her abundance of energy. For Race, keeping fit and prioritising wellbeing have always been natural parts of enjoying life. By the time Race was 20 years old, she was a professional dancer and first-degree karate blackbelt, having been awarded the title of Sensai.

Now in her 40s, Race has experienced what many people would consider a life less ordinary. Race speaks often of her profound gratitude that her life circumstances, though sometimes deeply testing, have allowed her the freedom to follow her inner voice, as well as the magnetism to explore all things that inspired her at a given time. Race feels blessed to have had the opportunity to form as a spirit in an authentic way — an opportunity that is afforded to so few of us.

With dance, theatre, music, martial arts and empathic healing as her foundation, Race was strongly moved by the creative freedom and self-identity she discovered while living in Sydney in the late 1990s and early 2000s. At that time, Race immersed herself in exploring Sydney's rich, unique queer arts and cultural underground. Fronting as a lead vocalist in live bands, and appearing in some of Australia's best-known theatrical performance art shows, Race grew comfortably and confidently into her own skin. Today, fire performance art is one of Race's main passions when it comes to fitness. Race views the dragon staff, a prop widely used in fire performance art, not only as a beautiful and hypnotic weapon but also as an avenue to rhythmic, transcendental meditation. Race believes that if each of us trusts and follows our talents and passions, as diverse or even contradictory as they sometimes appear, we can access a deeper level of soul serenity, emotional and mental clarity, as well as a sparkling and vibrant physical beauty and strength. By attaining this level of health and natural, primal fitness, we can change our lives for the better — and do it effortlessly.

FIT AND CHILLED OUT

Race has developed a simple, fun and powerful methodology to support people to awaken to the simplicity of living as their highest possible self — the Star Creature within each of us. Allow each puzzle piece of Race's methodology to gently guide you, and watch as the fittest, happiest, healthiest, most evolved and successful version of you emerges into its rightful place — shining bright at the centre of your life.

Synopsis

There are many evolved souls and highly sensitive people on this beautiful planet of ours. There are the deeply creative people and the ones who have always had the knowledge or desire to live true to themselves, in complete authenticity. Race has termed these people 'wholistic culturals'. Throughout their lifetime, wholistic culturals bounce back to their natural centre; they pick and choose what works for them; and they help keep the planet's energy growing and evolving in this wonderful, ever-progressing world.

Many wholistic culturals are 'Star Souls' — or old souls, to use a term that might be more familiar to many of us. Even at their happiest, many Star Souls feel an intuitive and intrinsic sense of deep restriction as they move through the world around them. This feeling of restriction, also referred to as a diluted spirit, stems from a build-up of stagnant energy. This burdensome energetic coating clings to many Star Souls, having been picked up from many sources over time. Those who suffer from a diluted spirit always experience an 'Aha!' moment once the condition is revealed to them. Suddenly, they are struck by a deep, instinctual feeling that they have been holding back (as a person, and even as a soul) from expressing the full power of their personalities — their innate goodness and vibrancy.

For these unique souls, intentional and full-hearted living demands that they unlock this energetic stuck-ness and stop stemming the tide of the magic that resides within them. To begin this journey, Star Souls must immediately and forcefully begin to tap into the actual essence of the highest possible version of themselves. That cliché of developing one's mind, body, and soul in order to attain self-actualisation? Turns out, it's true.

When a Star Soul lives their truth deliberately and fearlessly, sharing with the world the unmistakeable richness of their full personhood, the effects on their own life and those of the people around them are nothing short of miraculous. Simply put, Star Souls can change their life and their world by just existing and living their soul's true purpose. They can achieve deep soul relief and finally relax into themselves (not an easy feat for most Star Souls).

Wholistic fitness and wellbeing is the key for Star Souls to attain this mindset. Race has developed a simple, beautiful and potent methodology to support people to awaken to the effortlessness of living as their highest possible self. This person is your inner 'Star Creature' — the fittest, happiest, healthiest, most evolved and successful person you can possibly be. And the best part? The journey Race describes comes naturally to Star Souls, and the benefits of getting started on this road are instantaneous.

FIT
* AND *
CHILLED
OUT

THE ALTERNATIVE FITNESS CULTURE

RACE REDOMRA

FIT AND CHILLED OUT

This book is dedicated to Xena and Ella.

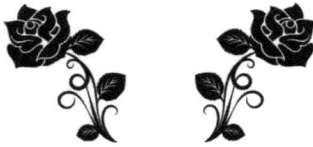

Contents

Introduction **15**

Chapter 1: Wholistic Culturals **17**

My five-step methodology 22

1. Cool Culture 23

2. Ultra-fit 24

3. Chilled-out 25

4. Clean Eating 25

5. Soul Serenity 26

Chapter 2: Black Sheep, Pink Sheep **27**

Remembering our true nature 27

Give me something that I can relate to 29

Do what you love and love what you do 33

Chapter 3: Finding Your Spiritual Identity Then Overcoming Obstacles **36**

Archetypes, totems, magical mythology, and finding your spiritual identity 36

Are you a Star Soul? 38

The top traits of an empath (or at least of this empath) 41

Self-sabotage 45

Procrastination and the 'Just do it' story 47

Time — where are you? 49

Money does not make the world go 'round 57

Chapter 4: Relax — The Hard Work Is Done **59**

More of a good thing 59

Meditations for the many 60

Chapter 5: Dare To Do It Outdoors **63**

Nature – she's free, and she's the best therapist 63

Ignore me, I'm just having a Zen moment 69

Contents

Chapter 6: Eat Real Food   **70**

Real-food tips   72

1. Graze   72

2. Buy what's in season   72

3. Never ever say the word 'salad' again   73

4. Eat clean   73

5. Eat more vego food   73

6. Prepare a Yummy Healthy Snacking Platter   74

7. Eat your largest meal earlier in the day   74

Tell me something that I don't already know   75

Chapter 7: Free Your Mind and the Rest Will Follow   **79**

Feed my hungry soul   79

Wholistic heart and soul — volunteering   84

Do you really live where you live?   84

Live and let live, love and let love   86

Synchronicity   86

Chapter 8: Magic Potions (Get Fit and Chilled-Out by Having Fun)   **88**

From diluted spirit to Star Creature   88

If it doesn't exist, create it   93

Chapter 9: Manifesto   **94**

Introduction

I am a wholistic fitness trainer and a first-degree black belt in martial arts and Zen meditation. From a young age, martial arts has provided a sense of security and grounding for me. I enjoy the self-discipline required, as well as the fact that martial arts are more than merely a physical pursuit. I have always had a strong intuitive feeling that what I could learn from martial arts was going to take me where I needed to be in this lifetime. However, I believe that the emphasis in modern martial arts practice has shifted from the spiritual to the physical. And as an empath (someone who is very sensitive to energy), I wanted to focus on the energetic and spiritual aspects of martial arts, not just the physical. My calling in life is to show you how liberating it can be to take control of your body and your health and fitness on your own terms.

In my time as a personal trainer, my clients, friends and family members have shared their feelings of frustration over the never-ending rollercoaster ride of health and fitness fads and phases. Some people do not relate to the mainstream health and fitness industry at all. I believe that the way in which health and fitness is marketed can be negative — even toxic — and that the industry can draw people into a web of consumerism and onto a non-stop treadmill of unachievable goals. Similarly, the beauty industry appears to target specific groups (especially women) in ways that can be extremely damaging and limiting.

I have found that for myself — and for my circles of creative people, artists, musicians, healers, and people who are into alternative therapies — mainstream ideas and images of fitness, health, beauty and sexiness do not resonate. The health and fitness industry offers quick-fix approaches, promising to help 'get your summer bikini body' or 'get your ripped abs for your wedding'. However, while this set course approach may work for some people, those of us who are freethinkers and who are more interested in alternative messages are unlikely to stick with these types of programmes. They are not designed for us.

I believe that the approach used by the mainstream health and fitness industry is not sustainable. With this in mind, I have made it my goal to find a methodology that will work for everyone in the longer term. My programmes are not willpower-focused but allow people to achieve the results they need without engaging in daily battles with their health and fitness. This is because, with the right approach, health and fitness come naturally. Having a healthy body and a healthy state of being is our natural state. Making improvements to your health and fitness should never be difficult or harmful.

Chapter 1 will take you through my methodology step by step. Throughout this book, I have included interviews with outstanding people who epitomise my health philosophy. I hope they will inspire and encourage you.

Chapter 1:

Wholistic Culturals

In 2008, I created an alternative fitness culture for like-minded people — people like you. Star Creatures Wholistic Fitness Retreats came about because I wanted to support my own communities in health and fitness: artists and creatives, people of diverse backgrounds, cultures and subcultures, LGBTI folks, old souls, the young at heart, and those who prefer alternative therapies. Through my programmes, my members and I develop healthy habits that we love, that fit in with who we are, and that are sustainable. Sustainable health and fitness practices lead to almost effortless and inevitable results — not just for six months, but for life.

My members are usually 'wholistic culturals'. I have coined this term to describe those who are not overly represented by mainstream cultures. In fact, wholistic culturals often make a conscious decision to seek non-mainstream sources of information. When it comes to shaping our ideologies and identities, we look to the richness and diversity of global teachings, ancient and new, to find what 'fits' right with us, aligning with our values and aspirations.

Wholistic culturals are able to see through the true intentions of the mass media. We do not identify with or relate to the type of information that is commonly presented to us and we know that the truth always prevails. Being individualists, wholistic culturals are often highly creative people, and are always freethinkers. We thrive in subcultures that support diversity, equality for all, and sound ethics. We need more than what is offered by mainstream information sources. For these reasons, I always urge the members that I support to look inward, trusting their own truth, wisdom, and intuition above all else.

The approach I've described so far is a good start to attaining health and fitness. However, in this era of selfies and social media, where narcissism is condoned and incentivised, there is a lot of confusion around this topic, especially among young people. Even wholistic culturals need something more than what's currently available, something they can love and find sustainable. So, I created and licensed a 5-step methodology that I guide my clients through. I have written this book because I want to share this methodology with as many people as possible, in order to equip them to achieve sustainable health, fitness and happiness that is more than just a fleeting fad or phase. My methods can transform you from feeling diluted in your spirit to becoming a Star Creature — which means that you are the fittest, healthiest version of yourself that you can be. And the best part of this approach? You can become a Star Creature in your own unique and quirky way — in a way that resonates deeply and meaningfully with your own truth.

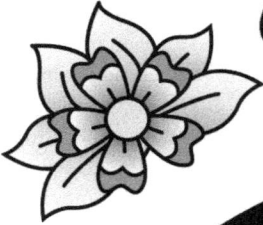

Interview
WITH

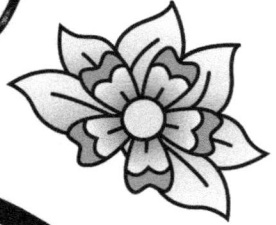

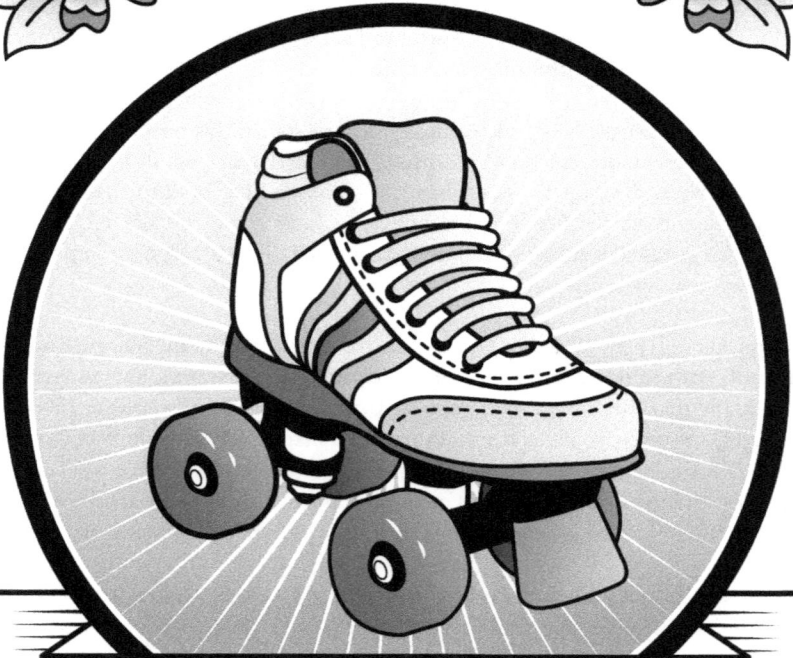

Robyn Soper

FIT AND CHILLED OUT

(AKA Great Bolz O'Fire, Sydney Roller Derby League and former Captain of the NSW/ACT Vagine Regime and the Beauty School Knockouts; Captain of Sydney University Freestyle Wrestling Team and NSW State Champion: Women's 63 kg)

Let's pause for a moment to read about how Robyn Soper got started in her field. You might not aspire to reach the same sporting heights as Robyn, but you'll doubtless be inspired by how she leveraged an activity she loved in order to bring herself great rewards in life.

- Race: Tell me a little bit about your story as a kid — the stuff you did that was active, like skating, gymnastics, etc. — into your teens and adulthood.

- Robyn: I was always a very busy child. I woke up at the crack [of dawn] and went to bed at sundown. I was made to do Physical Culture when I was nearly 5 and remember struggling to remember which [way was] left and which was right. My mother quickly realised I needed more action and whipped me out of that into gymnastics, which I spent the next 10 years doing. I was very flexible, and [my parents] had hoped I would be a contortionist when I grew up. I had 4 big brothers and sisters much older than me — they used to get … dropped off at the local roller rink while I had to wait in the car because I was too young. I think this [experience] left me determined to conquer what was inside [that rink]. As soon as I was old enough, I started lessons in artistic skating.

Then, when I'd completed all that, I did speed skating and only stopped to make way for gymnastics and high school. At around 8 years old I wished for gifts like a BMX bike, skateboard and weights. I used to do Aerobics Oz Style in front of the TV at 5 am but was so shy I never let anyone know and would always deny it if I got caught! I never got the weights as my mother thought them inappropriate [given my age], but I did get a silly, pink hand-me-down bike with streamers and spokey-dokeys and one of those plastic banana skateboards that are back in fashion now. It was the '80s and skateboarding was blowing up. I never changed [since that time]! As an adult, I now have my own gym, weights, lots of skateboards and a BMX.

- Race: What attracted you to the [roller derby] culture, and why did you feel like you would fit in?

- Robyn: I knew, with my skateboarding background and love of fierce, strong women, that roller derby would suit me. By the time the first league came to Sydney, my daughter was 1 year old, and I was ready to make time for myself to do something I enjoyed that was for fitness as much as making friends, having fun, and getting my life back. I had done speed and artistic roller skating as a child, so thought [roller derby] would come easily to me. Eventually, I found it did. But not without a lot of pain along the way!

- Race: Tell me about your own fitness/health transformations (times of being mega fit, and also times of slowing down) and what you still do [for fitness] that is second nature.

- Robyn: Before roller derby, I didn't have much endurance fitness at all and had always hated cross-country/endurance-style exercise like bike riding and running. In my 20s, I discovered yoga, which I fell deeply in love with. Being a flexible person, it all came to me very easily and I spent years doing yoga many times a week — all through my pregnancy and then mums-and-bubs yoga afterwards. I had never enjoyed team sports until I started roller derby. Being on a team meant you had to train to a schedule to keep your spot on that team. I liked the discipline and it really drove me to be better, get fitter and train harder to be the best.

The fittest I ever got was when I played roller derby. By the time I was selected to try out for the national team, I was doing 10 hours of exercise a week. A regular training week was 5–7 hours on skates and 3 hours off skates. I also realised that I could ride ramps in my quad skates because of my experience in a skatepark on a skateboard. It came very naturally to me and before long I was skating vert ramps and living out all my skateboarding dreams on quads. So, on top of the 10 hours' exercise [each week], I was also riding ramps twice a week at least or jam skating or street skating. The exercise was invisible as I was just having fun with my friends, learning tricks and living the life.

Then, four years into my derby career, I decided to give freestyle wrestling a go in the off-season. [Wrestling required] a different set of fitness altogether, using muscles I didn't use at all in derby. It hurt a lot, but I stuck at it and when the excitement of roller derby waned, I left to concentrate on [wrestling].

I transitioned from derby to full-time freestyle training with no break. I was worried that I would lose that level of fitness, so used the same theory of training I used with derby. I trained 4 times a week, and at [my] peak 6 times, doing weights and cardio in between open mat and technique lessons. Everyone thought I was mad, and I did eventually settle down a little. I see now that training less in the lead up to a comp helps you sustain your fight weight, sleep better and have more energy and mental stamina on the day. I took my first real break in 6 years this Christmas holidays, when I took 6 weeks off wrestling training. I still worked out 3–4 times a week; however, [I] took 2 full weeks off doing anything. I'm not sure that I did lose that 'derby fitness' in that time, but it was hard getting out of holiday mode and back into full-time training. I think my body needed [the rest], though, for sure.

- Race: Tell me about derby chicks' awesome fitness transformations. I especially love to hear about people giving up smoking, losing weight, building mega muscle, etc.

- Robyn: Roller derby used to be very popular with the bigger ladies — although they never stayed big for long after taking up the sport]! The beauty of an all-inclusive sport is that people who have never done any sort of exercise before sign-up like mad. One girl, who was [new to the sport], extremely overweight, and a very slow learner, stuck at it and ended up half her size and on the travel team. In the beginning, it was a party sport. Girls would train hard, then party hard — [there was] always a big group outside [the rink] smoking. We would have jelly wrestling at our Xmas party, and it was very wild. We really liked to let our hair down!

As the competitions got more serious, though, most people joined a gym, gave up smoking and stopped going to after parties. We went from [being] party girls in pretty outfits to serious athletes who spent their downtime in the gym or on-line watching derby games streamed from the [United States]. It certainly empowered a lot of women, [with] some going on to take up [mixed martial arts], boxing, and other serious sports.

- Race: Would you say your fitness and wellbeing is sustainable through your sports?

- Robyn: [At the moment], I'm starting … a new year of freestyle wrestling training. After 2 full years of learning, I think I still have another year before it will come naturally when I face off in competition.

[For wrestling], my cardio fitness needs to be extreme. A wrestling match goes for 2 x 3-minute rounds and is won by either points or pinning your opponent's shoulders to the mat for 3 seconds. For those 3-minute rounds, you are fighting for your life and using every muscle in your body. Keeping game-fit requires a certain amount of nutrition, cardio, technique, strength, and rest. I recently got a nutrition-extraction blender and have been substituting any snacks I have in the day with a veggie and fruit blend with lots of water.

[With this approach], I have found I have plenty of energy and have kept to my lightest weight without trying. I have a schedule that I ramp up towards a competition and [I] unwind after [a comp], making sure I give extra time to my family, who support me in all my goals. I try to schedule holidays throughout the year to give my body time to rest, heal, and most of all relax.

Roller derby used to take up 90% of my year. [In contrast], I love the freedom of doing an individual sport, where you put in as much as you want, when you want. I rarely roller skate these days and I find yoga too bloody Zen for my head space when I'm in full-on training mode for wrestling. I'm an all-or-nothing type of gal and who knows what I'll be doing next!

My
Five-Step
* Methodology *

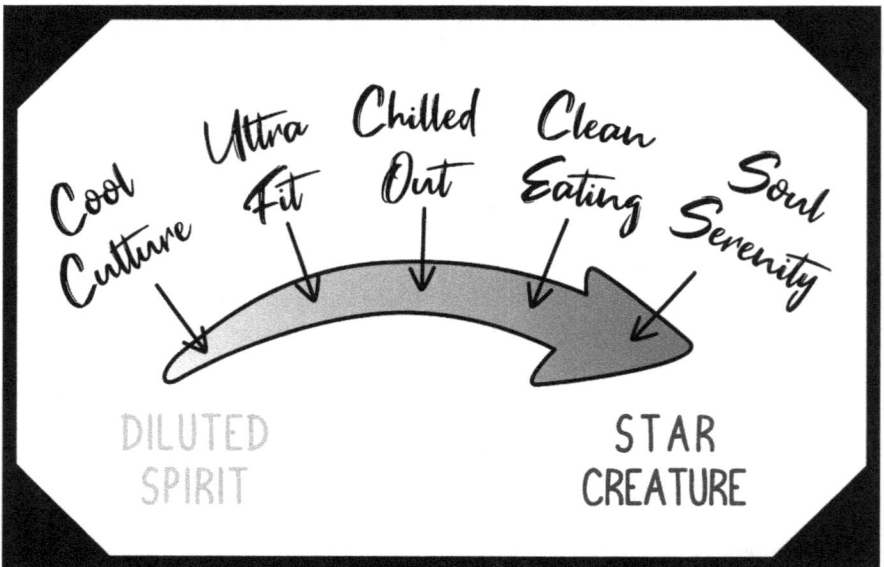

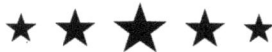

Cool Culture

Ultra Fit

Chilled Out

Clean Eating

Soul Serenity

DILUTED SPIRIT

STAR CREATURE

★ ★ ★ ★ ★

FIT AND CHILLED OUT

My 5-step approach to becoming a Star Creature

Becoming a 'Star Creature'

All the steps in my methodology are about balance. That's why I decided that we needed 5 pieces for this puzzle — that is, 5 steps for this methodology. Wholistic fitness is about your wellbeing as well as your fitness. To look like a bodybuilder, you must train 6 days a week, for at least 4 hours a day. That lifestyle is neither fun nor practical for most people. With only 24 hours in each day, most of us want to spend our time doing what we love with our family, our friends, and just living life.

Let's look at each of these steps one by one.

1. Cool Culture

The first step in my methodology is called 'Cool Culture'. This means connecting with like-minded people with whom you feel comfortable — a sense of shared identity and communion. These people are going to reciprocate support, be there for one another, and identify with being fit and healthy in a way that works and that feels right for them. Finding a way of identifying as a fit and healthy person will be different for everyone. But the main focus is on finding your higher self, your Star Creature — the person within you that is the fittest, healthiest, happiest, most heart-centred version of you.

Cool Culture is about putting yourself into the right environment with the right people. When I look at culture and subculture, I see people who set their own norms and values — people who connect with those they feel comfortable with and identify with. In any culture and subculture, and for artists and creative people, in particular, it can be difficult to connect with people who have the same interests and who also identify as being fit and healthy. I realised that we needed to put time and energy into thinking about the types of environments that we require in order to nurture our cultural and subcultural needs at the same time as we strengthen our identity as fit, healthy and positive people.

We may not have this positive culture in every aspect of our lives; we may only have it at work, for example. If we work in a healthy environment, and that is where our focus is, then that would be a good place to start a walking group or a tennis group or whatever it is that you want to do with people there. Even if you dislike gym culture or the idea of an early morning boot camp, it is possible to find fit and healthy cultures that you feel comfortable with and that include people you want to hang out with. A strong sense of self and connection is central in all of this.

2. Ultra-Fit

Ultra-fit is the second step of my methodology. Once you have sorted out your Cool Culture, Ultra-fit becomes more achievable. In Step 2, you'll discover what you like and enjoy about sustainable, wholistic health and fitness.

Look at where you are at in your life right now. Is there something missing in relation to your health and fitness? Is there something health and fitness-related that you have always wanted to do? Can you include it in your life?

It might help to reflect on what you loved doing when you were a child. A friend of mine was a child gymnast. Now, at the age of 45, she is rediscovering gymnastics. When you realise that you miss doing something that you used to love, it makes sense — and will feel natural and effortless — for you to return to that activity.

Put simply, Ultra-fitness means doing what we love. In the process, we improve our heart health, get rid of dangerous excess body fat, strengthen our muscles and improve our bone density. So swim, run, play hockey, bush walk, twirl fire, tap dance — find a way to do whatever floats your boat. Alternatively, learn something new, like cultural dance, hip hop, belly dancing or contact sports. When you find yourself missing these activities when you aren't doing them, you will no longer struggle with motivation.

In my methodology, Ultra-fit means being as fit as you want to be. I have clients who are elite athletes. Even for them, we are working on sustainability; we are working on strengthening the Cool Culture side of their health and fitness, so that they can continue doing what they love in different ways. For example, they might be a late-evening runner, but find that they do not particularly connect with the people that they are running with. In this scenario, we work on finding other enjoyable sports and activities with which they can augment their training. For people who want to be fit, we use this methodology to look at their goals in order to help them be the best that they can be at that point in their life.

3. Chilled-Out

The third step of my methodology, Chilled-out, represents every level of relaxation — from just literally chilling-out, having some siesta time, right through to deep relaxation practices. It is worth noting that once we embrace 'me' time in a guilt-free way, that downtime enables us to do our best healthy thinking.

I have lived in a number of big cities, and one of the problems that I frequently encountered was people with crazy schedules; even their dogs were on schedules, not to mention their children. It's good to have goals, to be motivated, to have schedules. That said, healthy, mindful living is not about scheduling your life right down to the last second, racing from work to meditation classes, all the while itemising the groceries that you have to pick up en route. That lifestyle just amounts to ticking a box or several boxes and simply saying, 'okay, done'. And by viewing meditation classes as just one more thing to check off on your to-do list, you'll miss out on many of the proven benefits of this transformational practice.

By loving our deeper relaxation practices, we not only improve our physical wellbeing — inevitably, we also become more cheerful and lovable, and we gain significant mental health improvements in the process.

4. Clean Eating

The fourth step of my methodology, Clean Eating, can mean different things depending on the context. Clean eating might mean eating food that's clean on our conscience, clean for the environment, clean nutritionally, or clean in terms of being free of genetically modified organisms and/or as organic as possible. Clean eating is not about eating less; it is about eating more.

By adopting my take on clean eating, we find ourselves eating more whole foods, more cruelty-free items, and more local, fresh and nutritious produce. I have an absolute ball creating meals for guests at my Star Creatures Wholistic Fitness Retreats. I source talented, clean-eating chefs who help me create food that tastes naughty but is delicious and nutritious. My members are jet-propelled with energy from food that is good for our bodies and for the planet.

5. Soul Serenity

The fifth step of my methodology is called Soul Serenity. Soul Serenity is an aspect of wellbeing that is often overlooked but is vital to tap into, especially in this soul-less day and age. Through Soul Serenity, we aim to engage in what some people call 'service'. Whether religious or non-religious, spiritual provision is the act of doing something good for another person. This can be working as a volunteer or going out into the world and doing what you know needs to be done, just for the love of it.

Soul Serenity also refers to genuine and random acts of kindness that help you and those around you to feel better. For example, it can mean simple things like making an extra sandwich and taking it to the homeless person that you have noticed a couple of times recently, or going to visit someone who may be considered an outsider by other family members, or hanging out with a mate who is depressed. It can also mean doing focused volunteer work that brings communities together.

Soul Serenity is about volunteering in ways that align with our passions in order to contribute in a way that is good for the heart and soul. It is about selfless giving, human-to-human and in-person, and can include activities like organising an important event, helping elderly neighbours, mentoring a young person, or even fostering a child.

Most of us apply some of these 5 steps to our lives. However, in order to become a true Star Creature, we need to embrace the whole 5-step methodology. We need to tune back into our true nature — the beautiful elements that we were born with, the things that we came to this lifetime and this moment with, the things that our very soul carried here. Chapter 2 will look more closely at how we can do this.

Chapter 2:

Black Sheep, Pink Sheep

Remembering our true nature

Some of us are lucky to have been able to stay connected to the different parts of our true nature throughout our lifetime. Some of us have become disconnected from our truth through life events, with intrinsic elements that we were born with becoming diluted or lost. Some of us have rediscovered those elements after a long, dormant slumber, often in the form of a spiritual awakening. I think that for most of us, our true, natural elements remain present throughout our lives. They just need to be brought back to life — to be rekindled.

Ever since childhood, I have known that acknowledging the things that make my soul happy generates a certain comfort and a strength of self within me. The child spirit arrives on Earth so very free. What better way to tap into complete authenticity than to revisit our childhoods, and in particular our pure nature? The mind and body can temporarily forget the rigours of adulthood; we can obtain a spiritual amnesia, returning to the free-spirited inclinations, attractions, curiosities and natural alignments that we had when we were children. In this process, I think that our innate soul knows when we are back on track.

We can initiate this process through a simple meditation. This meditation can be done as a one-off activity by sitting quietly and remembering. Or it can be performed regularly, as a series of remembering exercises that can be added to your practice after your body and mind have relaxed.

I have a couple of special memories that make me smile and remind me that I have always been a very sensitive soul. Being born a highly sensitive empath, I developed ways of allowing all the turbulent energy that I picked up around me to settle and to return me to a relaxed centre.

I can remember one of the bully kids who lived in the street next to my parents' place firing a BB gun at my neighbour's chickens from over the fence. He was laughing wildly, and not only at the chaos and fear that he had created among the chickens. He was also entertained by watching me cry and scream at him to stop. I had seen one chicken get hit and, being a typical empath, the image of the poor innocent creature being hurt would not leave my mind for days. It really upset me.

As a child, I had a number of natural sanctuaries or places of recovery where I could go to be alone and to simply process things. One of those places was the top of a very tall maple tree in our front yard. When I felt overwhelmed, I would often walk outside, climb up to my favourite branch and sit there. I don't remember how long I'd typically stay up there for, but my soul always seemed to know when I felt refreshed enough to come back down again.

As I write, I've just been reminded of another time when I retreated up into a tall tree when I was feeling overwhelmed. This time, though, I was 22, and hanging out at the house of a friend who had a few mates around. The next thing I knew, they had put on a horror movie. As an empath, I was so traumatised by what I saw and by the fact that my mates were watching violent and gruesome imagery for entertainment that I walked outside, climbed right to the top of the tree directly outside my friend's door, and remained up there for hours. Trees were clearly my 'safe place' back then. It's no surprise, then, that forests and the bush definitely remain a sanctuary for me today. I absolutely love them.

Throughout my childhood, another special place was the bushland at the bottom of my street. 'We're going down the bush!', my little bro and I would yell daily to a parent as the screen door slammed behind us. I must have yelled those words thousands of times during those years.

As a child, when I was feeling overwhelmed with the colourful assortment of chaos that could be going on around me at any moment, sometimes I would retreat to another favourite place. It was a stunning, tranquil creek, surrounded by willow trees and other wild, branched trees. The creek was often covered in water lilies and I always loved watching the array of beautiful native ducks that lived there. Here, I just was. I just existed. Totally simple, effortless, at peace.

What about you? What were your favourite places to retreat to? What were the nice things you did as a kid that your family or friends commented on? Were you the child who was always melting hearts by being thoughtful or compassionate? Did you adore animals? Try to remember in as much detail as you can. Can you recall the deep feelings of contentment you experienced when you first did something that made someone else happy? When recalling those moments, try to remember as clearly as possible the little details — the colours, the scents, the moods, the sounds and how people reacted to what you had done.

Think about the activities and the things that you really loved doing when you were a child. Did you enjoy focusing on a particular activity until it was completed? Were you dedicated? Or did you like loud and stimulating environments? Are your fondest memories of peaceful family picnics by a river or a boisterous day at the beach?

I believe that remembering these things and revisiting beautiful memories can benefit you in different ways. This process can be an amazing and effective relaxation exercise. It can also prompt you to think outside the box about a range of different and valuable topics, like 'Am I in the right job that suits my nature?', and 'What would be a wonderful holiday to allow me to rejuvenate from a stressful 6 months?'.

This exercise can also do amazing things for your identity and self-esteem. But the biggest benefit, in my view, is that this exercise simply reminds you that you are an individual, a perfect and unique soul, with your very own magical and spiritual nature. It illustrates to you that your uniqueness can shine brightly, whether you are a little kid, or buzzing, shining and sharing your presence with the world as a grown-up (or a big kid, as I prefer to say).

Give me something that I can relate to

Health, fitness and wellbeing — these are words used to describe a state of balance in your mind, body and soul. These words also refer to billion-dollar industries that target different aspects of health, fitness and wellbeing. Marketing to support these industries targets audiences by presenting a variety of stereotypical images that rarely represent or resonate with regular people. Nor do these images appeal to people who view themselves as being outside of the mainstream. Fortunately, there are a diverse range of individuals who embrace health, fitness and wellbeing on their own terms. I created my 5-Step Methodology with people like you in mind.

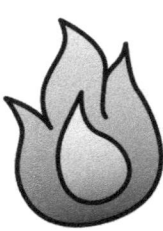 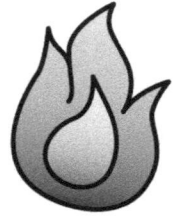

Interview
WITH

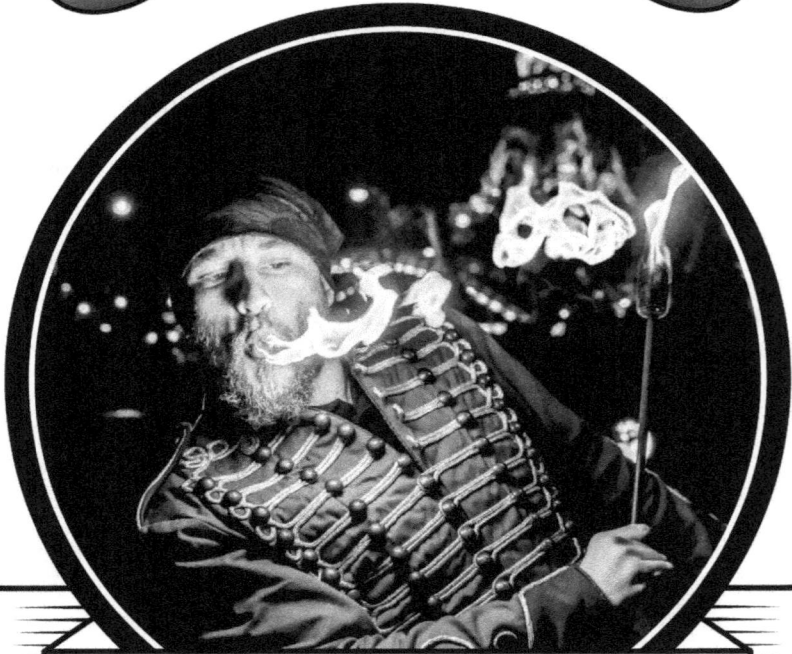

Shade Flamewater

✳ Two Questions ✳

FIT AND CHILLED OUT

Shade Flamewater is the founder of Flamewater Circus, a world-renowned fire circus from Sydney. Shade faced a major obstacle early in his life — an obstacle he found a creative way to overcome. You might never be (or want to be) a fire performer, but you can certainly be inspired by Shade's courage — and also make use of some of his great advice.

- Race: So, the first question I wanted to ask you is: can you just tell me the health benefits that you get from circus sports, and fire spinning in particular?

- Shade: Oh yeah, absolutely — strength, flexibility, hand-eye coordination with juggling, object manipulation, left-brain right-brain hemispherical cross over; [it's] good for your eyesight, good for your body, good for your brain.

- Race: And I would really love for you to share your story about your own personal health issues, specifically with osteoarthritis.

- Shade: Sure. From a real young age, I was just in my teens, late teens, when I got diagnosed with osteoarthritis. Had a lot of lingering knee injuries from when I was younger playing rugby and soccer. [The injuries] were really starting to act up. I was struggling to walk, get out of bed in the morning, and lo and behold I had osteoarthritis, which is uncommon for that age. [I had] a few years in my mid-20s where I was getting really depressed, didn't exercise, got overweight — and yeah, I was getting really unfit, unhealthy. I needed a lifestyle change.

I found a passion in circus sports, circus arts, juggling, staff spinning and fire spinning. What was great about it was it helped with low-intensity exercise, helped with strength and flexibility. I did a lot of yoga [and] stretching, which is great for osteoarthritis. [It helped] build up my muscle strength so I didn't ache so much, wasn't sore all the time, could get out of bed in the morning, that sort of stuff.

- Race: Fabulous. Low-impact exercise — that makes so much sense. Did you already have an interest in [circus sports], were you already practising a little bit?

- Shade: Yeah, certainly. When I was younger, I enjoyed some of the more kiddie-circus sports like yoyo, devil stick and the diabolo stick, little stilt walking things, that sort of stuff. As I got older, I got into the more professional side of things, a bit of acro-balance, a little bit of fire spinning. [That experience] definitely fed my hunger for [circus sports] and made me want to do it more.

- Race: So basically, you were able to get back into physical activities when you discovered you could put lots of time and energy into fire spinning. How much healthier and stronger and fitter do you feel [as a result of] doing this than if you weren't really doing much activity at all?

- Shade: Incredibly more so — I mean, like I said, I used to have problems getting out of bed in the morning, I was in that much pain, and now I run a fire circus and I'm going on a world tour. I say it's definitely beneficial!

- Race: That's so motivating for people to hear, absolutely. And I remember you saying too, when we were chatting, that your friends couldn't believe that you'd achieved this amazing international success. It must be a nice feeling to kind of prove people wrong!

- Shade: I can't really believe it myself. I do like to rub it in with my mother though. I like to say to her, 'I told you I'd become a famous fire spinner and you didn't believe me'. But aside from that, I'm just enjoying the success while I can. It's good to know that other people can be inspired to do [fire spinning] as well, 'cause it's a beautiful art form and it does keep you fit. It is good for you and I think more people should do it.

- Race: Definitely. [It's good for you] mentally, emotionally, and it is very meditative as well, isn't it?

- Shade: And very community-based. There's a lot of support from other circus artists around the world, [who'll] help teach and share and help you grow and learn more.

- Race: That's really important, being part of a community, but also contributing to community. People always feel safer as part of a group and if you can relate to a group that's doing awesome [stuff], that's going to keep you coming back, isn't it?

Also, I wanted to talk to you about a message that you might have for people that are embarking on, or are already established in, their alternative business. You were saying that you think that everybody can have success in their alternative business.

- Shade: Sure, well, I tell ya, I had a lot of struggle[s], especially earlier in the year with trying to keep my circus arts shop running. It was becoming very, very stressful, very difficult to figure out what my next move was. I got great advice from a lady that I knew; she is a Small Business Advisor, and she said: 'I've got two questions for you. First question is, *What do you really want?*'

I said to her I wanted to go travel the world
doing my art. She said, *'Okay, what's holding you back?'*. I said the shop was holding me back. And so I answered my own question as soon as I said that. It was like I had to get rid of the shop and within a week I managed to get rid of the shop and all my responsibilities tying me down, got rid of all my stuff and managed to line up a world tour, and now I have … what I want and I don't have the thing [that was] holding me back. Sometimes, the answer is really clear. Those two questions really helped me out.

- Race: So — what do you really want? and what's holding you back? There you go, two questions — simple. Sometimes, you can't beat simplicity.

Watch on Youtube Channel: Star Creatures Wholistic Fitness Retreats

FIT AND CHILLED OUT

Do what you love and love what you do

Go and grab a pen right now and write down (or type up) a few activities that you loved to do as a child — the things that you did often and without a second thought. Note down anything you did that involved physical activity, but only if you loved doing it. Ignore the activities that you quickly lost interest in, gave up completely or did not enjoy. Think, think, think, and more memories will pop up. Note them all down.

Here are some memories that I have recalled just now, off the top of my head. See if you can list more than I have. Take your time and think about it.
* Bushwalking close to my house
* Dancing in my lounge room to music videos
* Dance classes
* Karate classes
* Extra karate practice in the backyard or with a few team mates in a park
* Riding my bike to the beach
* Riding my bike to get from A to B
* Walking to the shops to do the entire shopping trip and walking it all home with my Nan
* Riding my horse to the beach or to a friend's house
* Swimming and diving in the surf for hours
* Jumping off my grandparents' wharf and swimming back to the steps, climbing back up to jump off again
* Climbing trees.

Select as many activities as you can — then, go and try them again! Schedule them so that you re-visit them over the next week and/or the weekend. Some activities will be very easy to incorporate into your life and others may require a bit of bravery, but it will be worth it, so go for it! Your soul will jump up and down, crying, 'Yes, Yes, Yes!'. The universe (or whatever or whoever your higher powers may be) will synch in and then scream, 'Well done!'. When you buzz and sparkle from the inside out, you emit an energy — a light — that other people pick up on. It is a part of human nature to feel and acknowledge positive energy. Everything needs light to grow, and when you are shining your light, you are weaving yourself directly into the energetic alchemy, the magic of the infectious and infamous 'good vibe'.

This step is imperative in tapping into becoming your star creature. Trust me on this one. Go and do it. Then wait and see how you feel.

Now it's time to make another list. Include all of the physical activities that you genuinely love doing or have loved doing as an adult. Include the subtler things that are active in any way, as well as practical fitness tips that you have picked up that fit well with your lifestyle. List all of the regular activities you do, as well as anything else that you have been too busy to do recently. Include all of these activities.

Here are a few of mine as a guide:
- Running on the beach
- My 30-minute express wholistic fitness session
- Push-ups and sit-ups on the beach
- Snorkelling
- Daytime music festivals and dancing for hours to beautiful beats or live music
- Martial arts under a huge tree in the park
- Burning incense and stretching in my lounge room first thing in the morning.

Hopefully, there will be a few activities on your second list that also appeared on your first list — activities that you love and have continued doing in some form throughout your life.

Here are a couple of easy-to-use tips that I have picked up from a variety of sources — including books, other personal trainers or colleagues, and television shows:
- Squeezing my abs when I am running, walking or sitting at my PC, to effortlessly improve core strength
- When walking on the beach for relaxation, walking on the soft sand to gain strengthening benefits effortlessly.

Keep referring to these lists, refreshing your mind regularly about these fun things to do. Remember, you know from experience that doing these things makes you feel good! Remind yourself of this fact, and over time you will find yourself doing them more often and looking forward to them. As an added bonus, you'll feel amazing, notice better self-image and body-image, and your fitness level will skyrocket once you have integrated your fun fitness stuff into your life and routine.

If you are already someone who enjoys keeping fit and getting your blood pumping, then drawing up this list will help you to tap into even more ideas.
If you are someone who isn't a massive fan of working up a sweat, you will be over the moon to re-discover activities that you used to enjoy.

According to the Australian Heart Foundation, we only need to do 30 minutes of moderate physical activity on most days of the week. Clearly, if you are doing activities that you love, you will be likely to average more than that amount naturally. It is never too late to start, and the Australian Heart Foundation has a free booklet that you can download from its website. You can download from its website. You can also request a printed copy within Australia. The booklet is packed with practical examples and is well worth taking a look at. Pick some cool activities from your lists and before you know

FIT AND CHILLED OUT

it, you can relax in the knowledge that your fitness requirements are simply and effort-lessly sorted, for life.

Chapter 3:

Finding Your Spiritual Identity
Then Overcoming Obstacles

Archetypes, totems, magical mythology, and finding your spiritual identity

I believe that there are numerous types of souls on this planet. Some of our beautiful Australian Aboriginal cultures (and there are many different ones scattered throughout the 'countries' of Australia) say that humans come from the stars and return home in between incarnations.

Personally, I have known for a long time that I am a Star Soul. This is a term that I have coined to describe the people among us who are, put simply, 'old souls'.

Many ancient and eternally wise cultures speak of people of the sky, people of the earth, and people with water energy. All of us have either animal totems or the four elemental associations of water, air, fire, or earth. Ancient mythology tells similar stories, as of course does the amazing world of archetypes, leading us into a more spiritually-connected kind of soul identity. For example, you may relate to the tale of Atlantis and have a deep knowledge that you are connected to the ocean. I have several beautiful and switched-on mates who talk about their associations with different magical themes, ranging from the sea to earth warriors, right through to the gentle forest elementals of pagan and Celtic beliefs.

I believe that it is important to take time to think about these things in order to help you find your spiritual identify. This identity may be completely separate from your religion (if you have one), or it may be intrinsically connected with it. Only you will know.

Human thinking, awareness and consciousness go in cycles around this stunning planet of ours. There is nothing 'out there' or 'different' about any of it. It is unbalanced to only focus on the conventional religions and belief systems that dominate mainstream cultures.

If you are reading this, I know that you, the freethinkers, black sheep, pink sheep, healers and intuitives, will understand exactly what I am saying. These ideas might especially resonate with you if you have been lucky enough to grow up in a proud and rich culture that subscribes to the deep and continuing celebration of soul evolution: reincarnation. If not, or if you are the type of person who loves the 'not knowing' and the mystery of it all … well, read on!

Highly sensitive people (HSPs), psychics, empaths, clairvoyants, indigo children, and intuitives are usually Star Souls. A term more widely used is simply 'old souls'.

I am an empath. I have not always known this, but I have always known that I had a freakishly accurate insight into exactly what makes people tick. When people looked into my eyes, and saw me looking into theirs, I could feel that they were either comfortable and drawn to me, or extremely uncomfortable — sometimes even scared. I was highly sensitive to my environment and would quickly either block other people's energy, protecting myself from it, or opening up and relaxing, depending on what kind of atmosphere and the type of people I was surrounded by.

What I came to realise is that I was sensitive to energy itself. I could feel it, scan it, react to it, read it, interpret it and experience a natural desire to 'move it' if it felt heavy.

As we all know, energy moves. We are made up of it. Every organic creature, being, and natural phenomenon is simply energy in a different form. (On that note, I love metaphysics — but we'll save that topic for another day). Children who are energetically sensitive can often process and transmute other people's negative energy with astounding effectiveness. I know that I could do this when I was a child.

Another way to describe negative energy is 'trapped' energy. In other words, trapped energy is energy that can't move, or that is stagnant, stale or stuck. When I was a child, some people loved it when I acted upon their negative energy. Others hated it. Sometimes people hated the process but loved me as an individual. Some people loved the cleansing effect but were unable to explain their outpourings of extreme emotions when they were in my company. And connecting with other peoples' trapped energy also had an effect on me.

I believe that children are still close to their original soul energy. As they grow into each incarnation, they are required to be a bit more 'involved' in their personality's energy. To put it simply, they need to learn the lessons that they are here to learn, in order to grow, to evolve, and then to leave when those lessons are completed.

Some of you will agree with this perspective, and some of you won't. And that is perfectly okay. We are all on our own individual paths, and I honour and respect your truth. The truth looks different from each of our billions of beautiful, unique, dragonfly angles.

Are you a Star Soul?

I believe that many of you who have been attracted to reading this book are Star Souls, and some of you already know it. If you haven't yet connected with your special and unique spiritual talent but have had an intuitive 'hit' in your extra senses from reading this information, then the chances are that you are indeed a Star Soul.

My parents both acknowledged that, from an early age, I was connected to extra senses and the spiritual world. When I was young, my mother took me to meet an amazing white witch healer, who taught only a small group, and I flourished under her tutelage. I learnt how to do more focused work, read auras and communicate with angels and spirit guides. I was given my first set of divination future-reading cards at a very young age. I loved to use those cards, especially in conjunction with psychometry. Psychometry is a simple technique where you hold a piece of jewellery belonging to someone and use it to tune into the energy of that person. For me, this process brought strong empathic sensations that I was able to interpret and transform for the person in question, giving them not only information about what was going on within their own being directly, but also the loving gift of healing.

Everyone is different, but empathic sensations I experienced included strong feelings about events (clairsentience) as well as flashing or emerging visions (clairvoyance). Occasionally, I would also receive whispers of useful information (clairaudience). Other types of star souls are indigo children, clairvoyants, intuitives, and HSPs.

As empaths and other Star Souls grow older, it can sometimes become harder to transmute, transform and recycle the darker, heavier, lower-vibrational energies that surround us. Often, these energies start getting stuck in our own bodies, manifesting as mysterious illnesses, aches and pains. It is often reported that HSPs will manifest energetically the direct illness of a loved one or person that they are in close proximity to. Spooky, isn't it? And yet, I know that this happens — because I have experienced it myself on numerous occasions.

In life, it is essential to identify your unique gifts and special spooky, freaky, or more subtle talents, so that you can then be aware of your deeper soul and the role that you play within your circles. In order to regain good health and wellbeing, this is even more essential if you have identified that something is wrong and that your power is being diffused.

This process is the first step to tapping into your Star Creature — your highest self. You can start by using the tools that you have available, including the simple 5-Step Methodology that I love to teach. Once you have some basic formulas to follow, you will be able to start living today as the best possible version of yourself. You can then get fit and healthy and stay that way with ease. You will stay cool, calm and collected as a result of attaining deep levels of relaxation on a regular basis. You will have that sparkle, that positive magic that makes you even more irresistible and lovable, and that makes people want to be around you. Once you are tuned into how easy it is to begin this journey, you'll find that your route unfolds before you quite effortlessly.

If you're a Star Soul, you have a lot of power that you can actually 'feel' contained within your being. Power that you know, on an intrinsic level, is very strong, and is energetically charged towards creating positive change. Star Souls know this about their energy, and at times they can be overwhelmed knowing that they hold a key to this type of power.

Star Souls reincarnate time and time again to evolve as quickly as they can in each lifetime, often choosing challenging spiritual journeys as a means to attain more growth in less time. Star Souls may also play a role in helping other people evolve by acting as a catalyst for change or growth. Star Souls are here to break cycles, creating and birthing new energies.

Some pioneers throughout history (and herstory!) were star souls. I believe that many celebrities, professional creatives, and other highly successful and hard-working freethinkers who have direct access to large groups of people through their positions of influence are Star Souls.

Entrepreneurs and founders, owners, or managers of alternative businesses and organisations may also be Star Souls. Many of these people eventually become known for creating change (and inevitably controversy) within their culture, community, or even in their families. At some stage in every Star Soul's journey, they become someone who creates 'evolution'. Regardless of whether Star Souls recognise this consciously or not, it becomes apparent in the level of success that they have achieved. Often, this evolution itself is precisely what is feared by the people around the Star Soul in question. Other people sense this force or power in the Star Soul, often resulting in the Star Soul being scapegoated. This happens because other people who are spiritually and emotionally rigid may find a Star Soul's presence deeply threatening. The success of a Star Soul in directly assisting the human spiritual evolution process can materialise in the pursuit of change. Star Souls eventually achieve a deep and humble feeling of personal success in all their realms of being, spiritually as well as emotionally. Nothing can beat complete soul serenity. Nope — nothing at all.

Key traits of Star Souls:

- Star Souls seem to choose a more challenging path in life. This path is chosen in the form of their 'contract' with their higher power in order to evolve as quickly as possible.

- Star Souls have very clear passions, usually holding a really special talent in these areas. They know, on an innate level, where they can make the most positive impact.

- Star Souls are drawn to things that are spiritual or philosophical, especially subjects that address the presence of 'a bigger picture' in life, and of our universe.

- Star Souls have an 'aura' or energy about them that, when charged in a positive way, appears to be incredibly infectious. They are highly aware of the positive power they can exude — an energy that leaves other people feeling amazing. Star Souls are carers and healers. Some are highly aware of their natural ability in this respect, and have chosen to work in caring or healing professions. Others are not aware of the level of healing they have to offer, but have an inkling that they have something special to share. This feeling often keeps Star Souls in an underlying state of searching for a higher purpose.

- Star Souls feel extreme guilt after displaying or processing their lower-vibrational energies (such as anger, jealousy and resentment) around other people. This tendency stems from their intuitive understanding of how powerful their auric field (or energy) actually is, and their knowledge that other people are deeply affected by their energy. Star Souls experience an overwhelming desire to either apologise or make up for this in their own way.

- Star Souls are usually extremely special individuals. Their way of communicating and expressing themselves is admired by others, who appreciate their genuineness and authenticity. However, new souls or people with a lot of heavy, dense energy or other problems can find Star Souls intimidating or may envy their ability to positively influence others.

- Star Souls have stages in life, whether childhood, adulthood or both, where vivid and very realistic dreams take place. Often, although these dreams are set in places or with people the Star Soul doesn't know in their current life, they experience second-nature familiarities during the course of the dream.

- Star Souls have an aura of 'wisdom' about them and people are drawn to them to help fix their problems or just to talk. However, Star Souls often have trouble finding friends, family or partners who reciprocate the same level of strength and care towards them. If Star Souls have other strong souls in their lives who can be genuine supportive shoulders to lean on through tough times, Star Souls will appreciate these rare connections and honour them with great respect and gratitude.

Do you think that you may be a Star Soul? Did you get that intuitive hit that resonated with you when you first read my words?

Unfortunately, there is another, darker aspect of being a Star Soul. I call it spirit dilution.

Has your Star Soul been diffused?

Listed below are the top signs of a Star Soul who has been diffused — that is, their spirit has become diluted. 'To diffuse' is defined as 'to make less brilliant; soften; or to make less intense; weaken'. If you have identified that you are a Star Soul and you are experiencing some of the symptoms below, there is a good chance that you are suffering from a diluted spirit:

- You have experienced stages in your life where you have felt as though you have an inner power that can't get too 'out of control'. You are fearful of coming across as being too much — too intense, too different from everyone else — when you fully express yourself.

- You are tired and drained by certain people, especially those who seem to sap your energy even when you have attempted to stop giving to them.

- You are aware of people who may feel the need to belittle you, draining your energy.

Spirit dilution is a common problem that can have dire effects on Star Souls, weakening drastically their chances of living out their full potential in life and, in particular, stunting their soul's evolutionary journey.

The top traits of an empath (or at least of this empath)

If the above discussion of what makes a Star Soul resonated with you, and now that I am supporting you as your wellbeing guide, you may be curious to read more about the particular type of Star Soul that I am: the empath. Empaths are extremely sensitive to energy. We have the special ability to detect it, analyse it, transmute and transform it.

Many of you Star Souls out there may find that you are empaths too. We are often drawn to each other.

I have gathered a lot of useful information over the years on what it means to be an empath and have incorporated some of the attributes into this section. Note that I have included only the elements that I relate to.

Remember that these are generalisations and that they may not always be obvious or apply to all empaths. Out of the hundreds and hundreds of traits that I have read, there have only ever been about 3 or 4 that do not apply to me. Other empaths may find that that is true for them also.

So, here goes ...

- We are free thinkers and free spirits. We like adventure, freedom and travel.

- We are drawn to healing, wholistic therapies, and all things metaphysical. Anything of a supernatural nature is of interest to us and we are not easily surprised or shocked. We are most likely to have had varying paranormal experiences throughout our lives. Near-death experiences and/or out-of-body experiences can catapult an unaware empath into the awakening period and provide the momentum for a journey of discovery. We frequently experience déjà vu and synchronicities. What may initially start as a feeling of 'Oh, what a coincidence' will lead to an understanding of synchronicities as an aspect of who we are. These experiences will become a welcomed and continually-expanding occurrence. As an understanding of self grows, the synchronicities become more fluent and free-flowing. They can promote a feeling of euphoria, as we identify with them and appreciate the connection to our empathic nature.

- We know stuff. It is a knowing that goes way beyond intuition or gut feelings. This gift becomes stronger the more attuned we are.

- We feel others' emotions and take them on as our own. This is a defining trait of empaths. Some of us feel the emotions of those nearby and others will feel emotions from those a vast distance away, or both. The more adept empath will know if someone is having bad thoughts about them, even from a great distance. We even know if people are lying to us (although some of us try not to focus on this because knowing a loved one is lying can be painful). We also know if someone is saying one thing to us but feeling or thinking another.

- We pick up sympathy pains, or physical symptoms of illness from other people, especially from those we are closest to.

- We always look out for the underdog: anyone who is suffering, in emotional pain or being bullied draws our immediate attention and compassion.

- We are quiet achievers.

- We are creative. From singing, dancing, acting, drawing or writing, we have a strong creative streak and a vivid imagination. The arts are chock-full of us! We are just as expressive with body language as with words, thoughts, and feelings.

- We love nature and animals. Being outdoors in nature is a must for empaths, and pets are an essential part of our life.

- You can often find us among volunteers. We love to work for the sheer love of it —especially with people and animals and for the environment.

- We love to daydream: We can stare into space for hours, in a world of our own, blissfully happy.

- We're great listeners. We won't talk about ourselves much, unless it is to someone we really trust. We love to learn and know about others and we care, genuinely and on a deep level.

- We strive for the truth. Anything untruthful feels plain wrong. This feeling becomes stronger when we discover our spiritual gifts and birthright. Linked to this trait, we are always looking for answers and knowledge. Unanswered questions can frustrate us, and we will seek confirmation if we have a knowing feeling about something. Sometimes this tendency leads to information overload.

- We are problem-solvers, thinkers, and students of all types of things.

- We often are vivid and/or lucid dreamers. Often, we feel as though our dreams are linked to our physical life somehow, and not just a jumble of nonsensical, irrelevant, meaningless images. From an early age, this curiosity will lead many of us to unravel some of the mysterious content of our dreams, connecting our interpretation to its relevance in our physical life. If not, we may be led to dream interpretations through other means.

- We have a broad interest in music to suit our expressive temperaments. Others may marvel at how we can listen to one style of music and then, within minutes, change to something entirely different. Lyrics within a song can have adverse, powerful effects on us, especially if they are relevant to a recent experience. In these moments, it is advisable for us to listen to music without lyrics, to avoid wreaking havoc on our emotions!

If most or all of the above points resonate with you, then you are most definitely an empath.

So, what are the downsides of being an empath?

- We tend to feel what is outside of us more than what is inside of us. This can cause us to ignore our own needs.

- Many of us would love to heal others but can end up turning away from being healers after qualifying (even though we have a natural ability for it), because we take on too much from the ones we are trying to heal.

- We find violence, cruelty or tragedy in any form (even fictional) unbearable. This aversion intensifies the more attuned we become. Eventually, empaths may find that they have to stop watching TV or reading newspapers altogether.

- Being in public places can overwhelm us. Places like shopping malls, supermarkets or stadiums where there are lots of people milling around can fill us with the turbulent emotions that are emanating from others.

- People want to offload their problems on us, even strangers. We can become a dumping ground for other peoples' problems if we're not careful.

- We're often tired. We get drained of energy, either from energy vampires or from taking on too much from others, which even sleep will not cure. Some of us get diagnosed with ME/CFS (myalgic encephalomyelitis or chronic fatigue syndrome).

- We crave solitude. We will go stir-crazy if we do not get enough quiet time. This is even obvious in empathic children.

- We get bored or distracted easily if not stimulated. Work, school and home life have to be kept interesting or we will switch off and end up daydreaming or doodling.

- We find it impossible to do things we do not enjoy. Doing things that we don't enjoy feels like living a lie. For this reason, many of us can get labelled as being lazy. But to force us to do something we dislike through guilt or labelling us as idle will only serve to make us unhappy.

- We abhor clutter. Clutter makes us feel weighed down and blocks the flow of energy, even when we may have been the person who allowed the clutter to build up in the first place.

- We attract narcissists! Unfortunately, narcissists like us. They like to use us as vessels with which to transform their endless stream of negative and stuck energy.

- We sense the energy of food. Many of us do not eat meat or poultry because we can feel the vibrations of the animal (especially if the animal suffered), even if we like the taste.

- We sometimes appear moody, shy, aloof, or disconnected. The face we show to the world is always our true face because we detest having to pretend to be happy when we're sad. This tendency makes working in the service industry, where service with a smile is de rigueur, very challenging for empaths!

Some empaths do not understand what is occurring within them. They may have no idea when they are feeling another person's emotions as their own and reflecting those feelings outwardly. They may feel confused as to how all can be well one moment, and yet they feel depressed and alone the next. The need to understand the possibilities of empath connection is a vital part of the empath's journey, both for themselves and for those around them.

How can you help an empath? Abandoning an empath when they feel emotional or, worse, if they feel that the 'whole truth' is not being told, is not the best choice. A simple return of empathic love, like listening and caring compassionately without bias, judgement and/ or condemnation, can instantly help put the empath in your life on the path to recovery.

If you are, in fact, a Star Soul, but with gifts that are different to an empath's, I hope that reading this section has inspired you to do some research to help you find your way in your spiritually-gifted role in the here and now.

The resources used in this section include:

- www.TheMindUnleashed.org

- www.spiritualunite.com/articles/30-traits-of-the-empaths-are-you-one

Self-sabotage

I'd much prefer to administer my own pain. But thanks anyway ... really.

Some years back, I wrote a song on a Celtic harp called 'Sabotage'. I have never per-formed it live, but I did record a cool version of it one day at home with just hip-hop beats and my vocals. The lyrics are as follows:

I know her now. Her face seems covered in grey. She said ... I don't want her now. I only want her when she's gone away. Sabotage. I'd much prefer to administer my own pain.

Each and every human being has an internal voice of self-sabotage that can attack when we are not at our best. Of course, people sabotage themselves for different and deep-seated reasons.

In this section, I hope to spark some thought space about how you can break the unpleasant sabotage cycle.

We all get held back through 'negative introjects'. Negative voices of the past can stem from other peoples' ill-placed words or comments, or our experiences. These can be traced back to childhood and to earlier familial experiences and hardships. As I sit here and acknowledge at this moment the traditional owners of the land where I write, thoughts fill my mind of the awful series of events that impacted upon Aboriginal people in Australia and in other parts of the world — experiences that are carried through time and through generations. Healing happens in its right time. I am privileged to know amazing human beings who have had deeply painful experiences, either personally or through experiences that have been carried down through generations. They have not only survived — they have thrived! Through expression, art, spiritual work and healing, these people have made their mark on the planet during their time here in ways that are nothing short of inspiring.

I was curious to know more about what holds people back when it comes to really getting consistency and sustainability in their fitness and wellbeing. I wanted to expand on ways to support my members in achieving this and getting off the rollercoaster of fitness fads and phases once and for all.

A beautiful friend of mine, who has become a member of Star Creatures and joined me on a mini-retreat, opened up to me about her own self-sabotage. She is an amazing, freethinking and inspiring woman, who works with disadvantaged communities as well as supporting those with disabilities (which I prefer to call all-abilities). Given that she is a very high achiever and hard worker, I was curious to hear what she had to say about self-sabotage. Despite her high levels of success in business as well as in the wider community, she confided in me that self-sabotage was one of her main blockages. She struggled with deep and hidden feelings of thinking that she did not have the right to make her health, fitness and wellbeing a top priority. She said that she put these things way down the bottom of her list of things she considered important. When she wasn't feeling in balance, ignoring her physical and mental health brought her into an even more severe imbalance. When she was feeling more motivated and positive, the truth rang very clear — a knowing that these things really were of the utmost importance.

When big stuff happens, hard stuff, real stuff, tough stuff, isn't it true that we should take a big deep breath and remember that our own health, as well as the health of our loved ones, should be our number one priority? Without good health, nothing else in our lives can flow and grow.

Human instinct is one of survival. Maybe this is why returning to my beloved ancient warrior practices has always felt like a blessing to me. Being able to share these practices with other people, with my own intuitive support style in place, is something that makes me feel humble, as well as relieved to know that I can help others. The warrior energy is the most powerful human force we can harness. Our 'hara' (our centre of life-force energy) can propel us through the flame, the darkness of the ashes and back up into light and healing. It is a simple, natural progression of energetic movement, no matter which corner of this beautiful universe of ours you join us from.

As an empath, I have had a tendency to unconsciously allow myself to be dragged into connections with people with very 'stuck' energy, all sorts of victim syndromes, and addictions. The more stuck the person's energy is, the more they have stuck to me! In the past, I have become very accustomed to the roles that have been projected onto me, and I have been side-tracked in life by every type of addict that you can imagine — drug addicts, alcoholics, workaholics, gamblers, narcissists and so on. I have attracted people who want me to process their negative energy for them, instead of doing the hard work themselves.

These days, I like to put my protective shield on, to expand my heart and to fight negativity with love. I feel love and understanding for those who have hurt me. They too have been hurt. They too have been damaged. It is up to all of us as individuals to stop sabotaging our own future, whether that is through blaming ourselves or blaming others. I can't begin to express how much I love and value the relationships I have built with people who love and respect me and who also take responsibility for their own problems. I believe that as a Star Creature, living the most evolved version of ourselves possible, we are able to take responsibility for ourselves. We can break negative cycles and create a new energy for ourselves, our friends and family, and for future genera-tions. I believe that this approach must start with basic sustainable health and fitness, positioned in complete balance with wholistic wellbeing.

Procrastination and the 'Just do it' story

When I was a young teenager, I started doing some modelling, acting and TV extra work. As my dad was an actor and was running theatre companies, I had a real interest in all things theatrical, including dance and singing.

As I got a bit older and started to make a living from the arts, the idea of having extra financial stability appealed to me. Even though the arts were fabulous, the work was seasonal and inconsistent. I got into fundraising for charities and found that I loved this line of work, as it gave my work in the arts a deeper meaning. My first fundraising job was for a lost dogs' home. I went on to have several part-time fundraising jobs in different areas of business and charity, but organisations that helped animals were my favourite.

When I was 18 years old, I had a phone-based job working within an ultra-dynamic small team. The manager was focused, business-minded, highly motivated and motivating to work for. He loved my work and he noticed that I had a great way with people. He quickly promoted me to a role where I was dealing with people face to face.

We had high-pressure bi-weekly meetings where we had to meet targets and undertake different types of training. Thinking back now, the team was way ahead of its time in this respect. The aim was to have a strong team, and the manager used money as a focus (dreams of money, earning lots of money) to motivate his staff. I wasn't interested in the money, but I liked the challenges that we were given.

By this stage, I had already achieved my first black belt in karate and was performing my first role as a sensei (a teacher). During this time, I also studied for and obtained my Travel Diploma. As my next step, I planned to focus on being graded for and awarded my full first-degree black belt in karate. I had trained very hard for this grading while commuting a long distance daily (to Sydney from the Central Coast) and working in my first full-time position, in a large wholesale tour company. I got up at 5 am every morning, went to training, got ready and was on the train by around 7 am. After work, I would arrive back to the Central Coast just in time for a couple of hours of karate training. I usually went to bed at around 10.30 pm. I learned early in life that you can't achieve big dreams and goals without outsmarting the human desire to procrastinate. I had multiple interests in life, and to reach goals in some of those interests did require self-discipline, especially in the highly focused world of martial arts.

Now, let's get back to the sales job part of the story. One day in a high-energy sales meeting, the manager asked us to contribute to an ideas board of motivational slogans that we could use. We were asked to dig deep, to identify thoughts we used to keep ourselves motivated. My suggestion came easily. It was a very short phrase that I had come up with years before, which was a simple mind trick or, put more accurately, a mental redirection and change of focus. This phrase had worked exceptionally well for me, as it brought me straight back to the fact that I was simply procrastinating around beginning a task or activity that I had already committed to completing.

When asked, I offered my phrase to the manager to add to the whiteboard. He looked at me wide-eyed momentarily and said, 'I like that one', before scribbling it down, circling it, and continuing to ask other team members the question.

At the next sales meeting, the manager had integrated my slogan and had added it to the top of all of our motivational material. I was happy that I had been able to share something useful with him, as well as the team. I found it strange that he had not acknowledged that the slogan had come from me. I took this lightly and had a bit of a giggle about it, as it simply illustrated to me that he did not have great ethics. Eventually, I moved on to bigger and better things, leaving behind the job, the team, and a bit of my energy.

Later down the track, I saw my slogan being used by a gigantic, iconic fitness company. I had mixed feelings, of which one was pride that I shared the same thought patterns as someone else who had suggested this term as a motivational marketing slogan that had been so successful. Another feeling was one of mystery and thinking about how the 'collective unconscious' works, with the same ideas in a million brains floating around the planet all at the same time. The other strong feeling was that of sadness, that little old me could work off a personal motivation strategy successfully, share it with others —but that the slogan could become accessible to everyone who could benefit from it globally only if someone else carried the message. The story I told myself was that the 'someone' in question was better, more successful and more powerful than me. It was a strange feeling, but one that I no longer suffer from in this amazing information age. I love nothing more than knowing that I can share my experience, wisdom and motivations with anyone who feels aligned to my thinking. In just one click, I can share my energy and the universe that is me with anyone who might benefit from it. I love knowing that I can also support my clients and retreat guests to get better at sharing with the world at large the unique and wonderful universe that is them.

By the way, my slogan was 'Just do it!' (and yes, this is a true story).

Time – where are you?

I believe that when we say, 'I can't find the time', it really means that the time is just hiding and needs to be 'found'.

You will be surprised by how much free time can be found when you look around. Even though we have identified that many of the activities that we love doing are good for us, we still need to give them top priority in our day-to-day lives.

These activities are so important for one simple reason: because our fitness and well-being must come first. We are the lucky ones who have learned how to have this magic potion of a fit body and serene mind, effortlessly and sustainably for life. We need to ensure that it is always at the top of our lists. As we all know well, a fit, healthy and happy you makes a much better partner, parent, professional or friend. The key is to get good at simple time management. To this end, you can use a time-management schedule. This can be as basic as one that you scribble down and then just keep in your mind. Simply dedicate certain days of the week to certain activities.

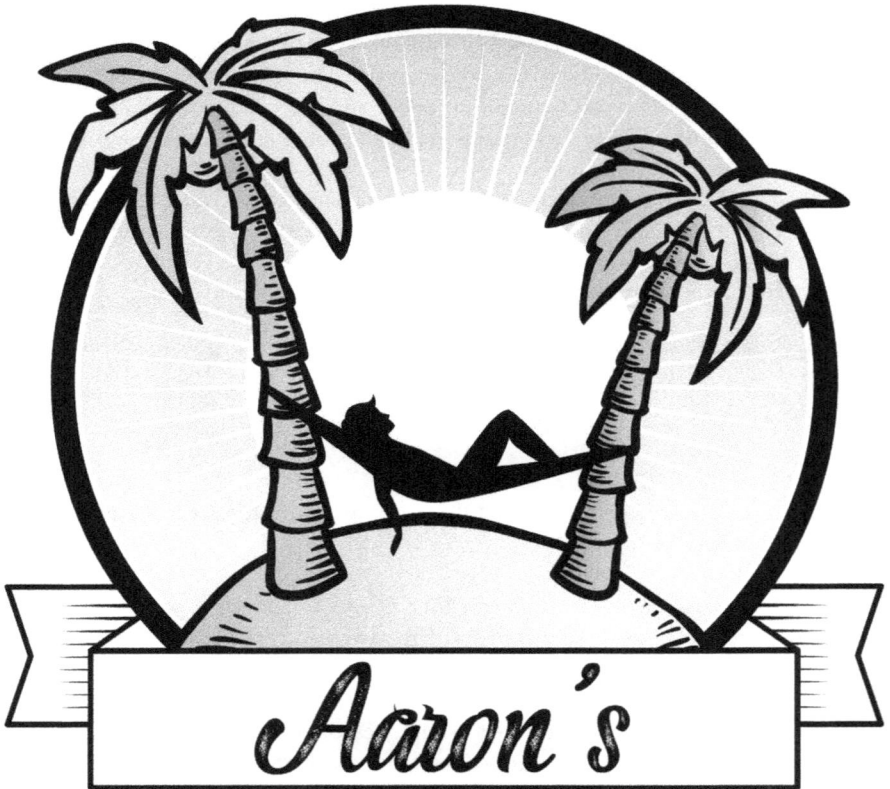

Aaron's

* *time-management* *

P L A N

FIT AND CHILLED OUT

Here is a good example of a basic time-management plan. Aaron wants to improve his cardiovascular health, drop some body fat, and spend more time in nature and serenity. This is his plan.

Every Saturday and Sunday, I used to get up and make a coffee and then drive to the shop and buy the paper and some groceries.

Instead, I now start weekend days by chucking on my running shoes and backpack and heading towards my favourite place, the botanical gardens. As I run or fast walk through the gardens, I breathe in deeply the scent of my favourite flowers as I take a detour through the rose garden. This always gives me an emotional lift and I feel really happy.

On the way back, I grab the paper and load the groceries into my pack before taking my time walking up the hill to my home. I then enjoy a gigantic bottle of water, a refreshing shower, a chilled-out read — and I relish every drop of my cup of coffee. I feel successful knowing that I have completed 2 hours of fitness activity, effortlessly, and that I loved every second of it.

I was a skater kid and was pretty good at it. I realised that I would be a pretty cool 50-year-old if I could skateboard again, so every weekday I now skateboard to work. I was a bit wobbly for the first couple of days, but now I'm cranking out all my old tricks. I love seeing kids do a double take and putting a smile on the faces of the commuters.

On most weekdays, I stop off at the local Buddhist centre on the way home for free guided meditation. I really miss it when I don't make it. It keeps me in balance and everyone around me has noticed the difference.

Since I've been doing this, I barely recognise myself when I look in the mirror. I see the fit young bloke that I used to be looking back at me and I love it. Everyone says that I am much nicer to be around. I am more positive, and I am having heaps more fun with my partner.

Let's look at this schedule:

- 4 hours per week running/walking
- 5 hours per week skateboarding
- 3 hours meditation

Aaron's fitness and wellbeing requirements are covered. Done.

This casual approach will not suit everyone, and more detailed methods and systems are always an option. If you are very busy, as many of us are, and you need intensive structures and a proper schedule, then it is likely that you already have a time-management system in place. Find an approach that suits your needs, and you'll love the feeling of knowing that you can fit in everything that's important to you. And you really can fit it all in! You can even schedule your days off, afternoons off, and small free chunks of time that pop up here and there. Identify those times, make the most of them, and you'll appreciate them so very deeply.

There is a way to manage time effectively to suit everyone. I write up my own regular weekly time schedule in my smartphone notes, and when there is a change, I look closely at how I can shift the time around to suit. If I want to visit a friend or do something random, I can look at when I have 'free time'. I find myself running down to the beach if I am going down there for a swim anyway. I might go to my favourite alternative dance class on a day off. And I love it.

Effective time management might be as simple as writing or typing something like this:

Monday	Morning off. 30 min weights workout and meditation. Workday 2–10 pm.
Tuesday:	Beach run. Fruit and veg shop. Workday 11 am–7 pm. Spiritual practice.
Wednesday:	Domestic Goddess (house cleaning). Bushland jog and picnic lunch. Work day 1–10 pm.
Thursday:	30 min weights workout and meditation. Workday 12–6 pm
Friday:	Day off.
Saturday:	Day off.
Sunday:	Morning off, then workday 1–8 pm.

Alternatively, you can use your calendar, a time-management app on your smartphone, or one of the free time-management templates that you can download online. Managing your time can be as basic or as defined as you need it to be. It is up to you so make time management suit you, so that it feels good and you know that your schedule is sorted.

I like to fool around and announce to those close to me that 'I'm on holidays'. When they look at me in confusion, knowing that I have a full week ahead of me, I cheekily add 'until tomorrow morning'. When your activity and relaxation needs are met as a natural part of your routine, your mind can be clear and present every single time you have even a microscopic amount of time off. This is true serenity. With this approach, you can be completely in the moment. Even just a few hours off at night to watch a movie or hang out with your partner or kids, being completely present and relaxed with them, is true bliss. And doing this will nurture all of your relationships, including your intimate ones. Your presence, without being distracted by the guilt of 'I should be doing this or that' will be met with appreciation by everyone around you (and by you especially). When you give yourself permission to truly enjoy your weekend, your downtime, or your holiday time, you are just so much more present in the rest of your life. Trust me on this one again, my stars. It is truly good vibes all around.

The magical and relieving part of tapping into your authentic active soul is that if something pops up that absolutely prevents you from doing your fitness or wellbeing practice that day, your natural desire will be to pick it up again because you will miss it deeply and you will flip back into action the next day. If you are truly forced to miss out, it is not the end of the world. There is no risk of dropping out completely because this is not a fitness or wellbeing fad or phase like those that you may have experienced in the past. These interests and pursuits come directly from you and are a part of you — a part of your life that you love, no less. You feel amazing when you do these activities, and they keep your body looking and feeling strong. They keep your mental, emotional and spiritual self on track, allowing you to sparkle and shine like the true Star Creature you are — your highest soul self.

Interview
WITH

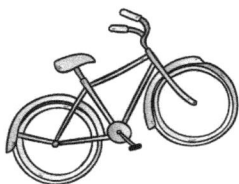

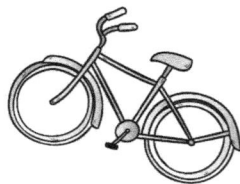

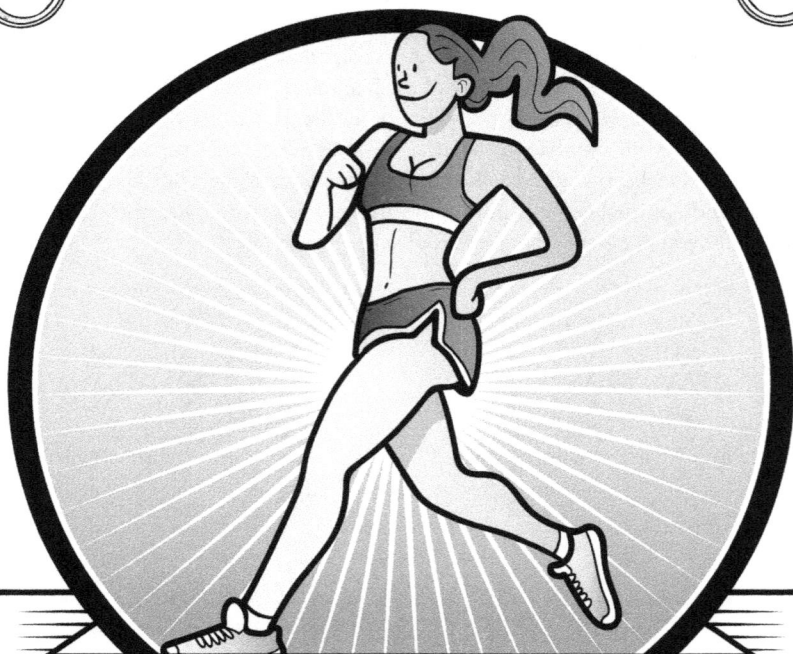

Kate Strong

* 2014 World Champion in Long Distance Triathlon *

FIT AND CHILLED OUT

The following interview is a true story about someone who realised, through trial and error, that they desired more from life than worldly acclaim in their chosen sport.

- Race: I'm really looking forward to sharing your story with the audience because it's such a fabulous story, and the way we originally connected was you telling me about that amazing turnaround in your career. If you could share that with everyone, that would be wonderful.

- Kate: Great. In 2012, I was a regular girl living a regular life, ticking the boxes of society. We all know what that feels like —should have a job, should have a boyfriend, should get a car and house and a mortgage and all that good stuff we're sold … [But] I realised I was existing and not living. So I chose to do what I loved. I lived in the Blue Mountains of [New South Wales] at the time, so I started to run, reconnect with nature and myself. Running took me to the swimming pool, and also took me to my bicycle. [The] natural [progression] was towards triathlon, [in] which I swim, cycle, [and] run regularly, by myself and in competitions. I won my second [triathlon] and was crowned National Champion for my age in Australia. So, 11 months after my first triathlon, I'm flying to China, where I compete for Australia — and I win that too, which earned me my title of World Champion.

- Race: Awesome. That's so good.

- Kate: I was pretty stoked.

- Race: I can imagine. So I'd love to hear about what happened that night you had your 'epiphany'.

- Kate: Sure. Once I started to train by myself, I realised it was much easier with a coach, someone to protect me from injury as much as make sure I got the best out of my body, and I did recruit a coach to write my programme. But I realised the training was sucking up my life. Basically, if I have to be dramatic about it, I felt regimented. You have to get up at this time, eat at this time, your body is secondary. I was disconnecting from the journey. And the journey for me was life. It's not all about the accolades.

One night, in a state of rebellion, I had an argument with my coach. I was up too late because the rule was 9.30 [pm] to bed. I'm 36, not a junior, so I grabbed my head torch and sleeping bag and just ran, ran through the forest. I ran using the head torch for the ground but also the moon to light the way to the sandstone cliff edge, where I fell asleep. I woke up to this glorious sunrise and it just reminded me that life is about connecting to your body, yourself and your journey.

Yes, it's nice to get external acknowledgements, but that's not why we do this. This is what it's all about. So, I listened to my heart and I listened to my body, and I still swim, cycle, and run — and I always do it with a smile.

- Race: That's just amazing, and what happened? What were the first changes that you put into place when you decided that you were in charge of your body?

- Kate: I chose to listen to myself. The alarm clock is not set each morning. If my body needs a little sleep it sleeps, if it wakes up at 4 or 5 in the morning that's okay. I eat when I'm hungry, not when the alarm goes off again. I'm blessed that I do work for myself. I am much more intuitive. If I'm tired, I sleep. If I'm awake, I do things, and I'm getting great results [with this approach]. I feel healthier and happier. My mood swings have lessened too.

- Race: And you look amazing, you look so beautiful, so vibrant. I can see in your aura and in your eyes that you're on the right path for where you are meant to be. Could I also ask you what would be your top tip in terms of sustainability, keeping true to the love of what you do for your body?

- Kate: It is a fine balance to listen to your body and rest or just be lazy, because our bodies love to relax and when you train for mainstream sports you do put the hours in.

One question I consistently ask myself is, 'Can it get any better than this?'. If I'm having a bad day, it's a great question to pick you up and still acknowledge that good things happen, if that's the only positive that you can see. But it also pushes me to ensure I'm being honest with my body and I'm not just using the excuse of pain [in my] muscles to stop the training session.

- Race: That's a great tip, thank you. I think so many people will get so much out of that [concept]. It's really, really important to stay in balance, and the more in balance we are, the more successful we can be. [You and I are] certainly like-minded in those ways.

Watch on Youtube Channel: Star Creatures Wholistic Fitness Retreats

FIT AND CHILLED OUT

Money does not make the world go 'round

This is an arguable point that I am making, and I understand that completely. The point that I want to make is that people often rely too much on money to provide things that could be done differently or even for free. Living every day as a Star Creature and enjoying your fitness and wellbeing is one of these examples. It is also very cool to know that you do not have to rely on anything material to have serenity. As long as the sun is still shining, the moon is still glowing, and the world is still spinning, we can all have health, peace and fun in our lives.

I have heard people say that they can't afford to renew their gym membership, and that the gym has become a bit of a white elephant anyway because they lost interest and motivation after a few months. If you happen to be a person who loves using the gym as part of your fitness practice, then you will find that it has already become a sustainable part of your life. You have been going regularly for a long time. In your case, I am sure that you will regard your membership fees as a priority for you and budget for them accordingly.

The same goes for any ongoing sports or activity fees for the things that you love doing. Paying for these things becomes just as important as buying food — and so it should be. It is an investment in your health, fitness and wellbeing.

It is worth pointing out that no matter where you live in the world, there are thousands of completely free activities for fitness and relaxation to choose from that are ultra-cool.

Here are some activities that I can jot down off the top of my head:

- Sightseeing walks in your own city
- A long bubble bath with beautiful music and incense
- Joining a dragon boat racing team
- Quietly observing your surroundings and other Zen-based meditation
- Social rockabilly and rock-and-roll dance groups
- Social community-run groups
- Skateboarding, rollerblading, and skating
- Chanting and meditation groups
- Indoor sports like basketball, volleyball, roller-derby teams — if you're a team player, the list goes on
- Night-time city-lights pushbike rides across your favourite bridges
- Swimming and surfing
- Snorkelling
- Burning aromatherapy oils
- Volunteering as a community communal gardener.

You can find ways to participate in many of these activities via the websites of community and online meetup groups. I always like to remind people that if you can't find a free group that you would like to join, you can start one of your own! Some time ago, I started a free community hiking group and made friends that I hung out with for years afterwards.

Some workshops and short courses may require an initial financial outlay, but they will offer subsequent benefits as you will have another activity that you can embrace and love for the rest of your life. That is very valuable in the long run. Feedback from guests that have attended my Wholistic Fitness Retreats verifies this: they have told me that they've been able to apply what they learned at the retreat to their daily lives. That was one of the main reasons that I created the retreats in the first place. I wanted to share with people all over the world that attaining lifelong health, fitness and wellbeing need not be constant sources of stress or expense.

There are so many different activities to choose from that will benefit your physical fitness as well as your emotional and spiritual wellbeing. Examples include:

- Deep-sea ocean diving
- Rock climbing
- Dance classes where you can learn hip-hop, flamenco or even breakdancing
- Tai Chi
- Surfing.

Chapter 4:

Relax – The Hard Work is Done

More of a good thing

Once you have embraced my encouragement to find fun in fitness, exactly the same principles apply to relaxation activities. It is very easy for hard-working, successful people to forget how important relaxation actually is.

Even from purely a productivity perspective, by incorporating regular breaks in the day, week and month, you will be more charged and powered up. More work gets done. The work you do gets done better. You are more switched on, more balanced, which of course results in your being more productive.

Let's also take a moment here to acknowledge the importance of relaxation on a mind-body-spirit level too. Relaxation is extremely important, and we all know the necessity of getting enough rest. You might already know about the positive effects of adequate relaxation in this respect, recognising how your health is improved by balancing things like stress and hormone levels.

Human beings need to relax. We need to enjoy life, to take time to stop and smell the roses, to have a good meal and a long lazy night full of laughs with friends, or to watch a movie. Whatever 'your thing' is, do it to relax more often. Take some time right now to make a mental list of all of the things that take you to the point of deep, healthy relaxation. I believe that this needs to be put on the high priority list. It is an important part of balancing our health — hugely important. And how fabulous that something that is so important also feels so good! Relaxing feels good because it is like being thirsty and finally getting that big drink of water. Take pleasure in making the time to relax on a regular basis.

When I was a vocalist in bands, being a typical artist, I was always busy with lots of different creative projects going on at once — band jamming, sweating it out in rehearsals, making costumes, and of course performing live. All of this was very time-consuming, but I loved it, so it was a worthwhile priority in my life. I was living in a remote part of Sydney, inside the Royal National Park. I had to write some new lyrics for a beautiful piece of music that my guitarist had written. I had a deadline of the next night, when we would meet to structure our new songs. I remember clearly that this was the night that it hit me that there were many things that I had taken on in my life because I loved doing them, but also knew that I needed to do them to feel fulfilled in my life. Instead of viewing the deadline as a stressor, I realised that I could tap back into the nature of my work, and the reason that I loved doing it. I remember thinking, 'This doesn't have to be yet another thing to do'. Although I was exhausted, I realised that, in addition to producing something that was needed from me, this process could be a relaxing and beautiful chill-out time.

I took a long hot shower and anointed myself in the most nurturing aromatherapy oil combination that I could create. I was using a lot of grounding cedarwood at the time, with a positive and light mix of citrus, usually bergamot oil. I mixed it with organic coconut oil and rubbed it into the palms of my hands. I breathed deeply as I pressed my hands against my chest, then my forehead, and then on top of my head as I took in the therapeutic and delicious scents.

I then took a walk to a tiny, unoccupied beach and into the forest, where there was a trail that led to ancient Aboriginal ground with carvings 30,000 years old. I sat and tuned into the sound of the black cockatoos that screeched and sung around me. I felt alive and relaxed. Reminding myself that I had chosen this path, I used my passion to propel me into being productive. I went into a Zen-style transcendental meditation and allowed my spirit to rise to a very high vibration and connect with my surroundings. By the time I made it to the carvings and sat down to go deeper into my meditation, the words for my song were emerging clearly. The vocal melody came through too and, before I knew it, I had a song. I was able to spend the last part of my meditation quietly singing my song, in a similar way to how some people use a chant in meditation. This song was born from my connecting right in deeply and allowing myself to fully relax and open up. On the way home, I lay on the beach for a few minutes watching the moon reflecting on the gentle waves, and feeling a profound sense of relaxation, satisfaction and serenity.

The next day in the rehearsal room, the song came together in our heavy industrial-style rock band. The song ended up being an intense, highly melodic but very slow and moving journey into the things that I felt and saw during the walk that night. I titled the song 'Ngaora', which is the traditional Dharawal name for 'black cockatoo'. One of my coolest memories from my rock-band days was performing the song on a live music-boat cruise when our band headlined. I loved watching people dance and get lost in the moment, as I described the sandy trail, the enchanted bush forest, the hundreds of beautiful, cross-patterned spiders swaying gently in their webs, protecting me under the glowing sky as I made my way to visit an ancient and magical place.

Meditations for the many

For some, the word meditation evokes the image of a solitary yogi or monk sitting on top of a giant mountain. A mind completely empty of thought and activity. Total stillness. Total bliss.

FIT AND CHILLED OUT

Totally unobtainable for the average person.

Often, in social or professional settings, people say to me: 'I would love to be able to meditate, but I just can't sit still and quieten my mind'.

This is a common problem, partly because many busy and ambitious people are mentally active, especially creative types.

Meditation can have many meanings, but it is essentially the practice of any healthy activity that can take your mind into a different state, a state that has wellbeing benefits. It may be an activity that gets your mind into a relaxed but very focused state that may help you to get an answer to an important question. It may be a practice where you simply sit and 'feel' your current emotional state and observe your breathing until you find that you are in a happier and relaxed state.

Having a background in Zen, I am naturally drawn to the beautiful and simple practices that are offered within this ancient philosophy. As I mentioned previously, observing nature and our connection to it has inspired ancient meditations that have originated from across the world.

One of my favourite parts of hosting retreats for my Star Creatures is guiding them through beautiful healing and rejuvenating meditations. I really do love doing this. I also like to record guided meditations and make them available for everyone to access on my YouTube channel. The awesome thing is that any meditation that takes your fancy is a search, click, watch or listen away.

Here are a few examples:

- **Zen Walking Meditation:** Involves simply tuning-in to your posture, your body, and particularly your movement. Each step becomes part of a (surprisingly relaxing) rhythm.

- **Buddhist Stillness Meditation:** This practice involves sitting still and in a quiet place. You may focus on one thing, like the song of a nearby bird, or the movement of the clouds in the sky. Whenever your mind starts to trail away from the meditation, you gently bring it back to the object.

- **Musical Journey:** I like to use headphones, burn incense or oil and light candles. Lie down and close your eyes, then let the music take you deep into another world. Sometimes I use meditation music, but I also use Bjork, John Lennon, Sia, Iggy Pop or heavy melodic rock. It doesn't matter what it is, as long as you can get lost in it.

- **Positive Visualisation:** This is a favourite with my friends and guests, and I love doing this meditation as well as guiding it. You can use it to focus on manifesting a positive outcome to a worrying situation, or as a healthy and ultra-positive relaxation escapism. Your imagination is completely private. It is owned by you and you only. You can go anywhere you want to go. Dream, dream, dream. Dreamtime, manifestation, magic, bliss, Zion, Heaven, Nirvana. It is yours.

There is no right or wrong way to meditate. The different methods are what they are and any meditation, no matter how deep you go, is good for you.

Chapter 5:

Dare To Do It Outdoors

Nature – she's free, and she's the best therapist

Everyone has a different way of relaxing on this beautiful planet of ours.

I have like-minded friends who absolutely need to be outdoors often.

I also know people who weren't raised to enjoy the outdoors, who aren't particularly into it, and may even have fears about it.

In my experience, and underpinning what I teach my students and guests, nature is an incredible healing therapy as well as a good leveller and natural reminder that we are all just tiny specks of sand in an unfathomable universe. This idea doesn't even need to be intellectualised. We do not need to think about that point for it to work.

When we are able to immerse ourselves in the bigger picture of the natural world around us, we become reattuned to our simple and instinctive sense that our day-to-day woes are pretty meaningless. Nature. The ocean, the trees, the sky, the stars, the fields, the snow and ice. Whatever it is, it is powerful, real, and each and every environment is not only a force to be reckoned with but a picturesque reminder that things change naturally.

No situation can ever stay exactly the same.

The tree that we lay under to read is getting bigger. It is growing as we lay there. It has a time and space code that is not detectable to the human eye. But we know that it is growing, right?

The ice will melt, and the seeds are in the process of sprouting, all without you or me having to 'do' or control anything. What an awesome feeling to know that if we just sit still, observe and trust in chaos, order will come! Change will come, too, in exactly its right time.

Ancient Zen meditations allow us to tune into nature to calm the mind, body and soul. In ancient cultures, meditation not only involves looking inward but looking outward to nature and, put simply, 'making the connection', whether on a lawn or in the wilderness. For those who are nature-shy or time-poor, sitting on a manicured lawn in springtime, on a rug with a hot cuppa can be deeply relaxing. Magic in nature is found all around us, even in the cities and suburbs. Anyone can take time out of the day to just sit and watch. As you sip your tea, you can close your eyes and listen in to the harmonies of the birds, which you may not have noticed until now. When you open your eyes, everything in the garden looks so bright and animated. The butterflies seems to be dancing just for you. You may spend a whole half-hour watching a spider re-weaving its web after a storm, sparking you to make a connection. Perhaps you are re-spinning the web of your life, creating your new future of dreams after a big life storm?

Regardless of whether you are camping and living and breathing nature for days on end or are taking a few minutes out of your busy life to unwind, tuning-in to nature works. It relaxes, revives, stimulates and recharges you. Whatever your needs are, being in nature just works — as everything in nature does.

Stargazing works. I love imagining how many human beings have stared up at the same stars that I'm looking at, over how many thousands of years.

Have you ever sat outside on a comfy chair, tired and almost ready for bed, or lay on your back in your yard and just taken a deep breath of relief and simply looked up? It is one of my favourite things to do.

I absolutely love letting my eyes go out of focus and watching for shooting stars. Once I am in 'star mode', I can start to see the different coloured glows that each star or planet has. Some are so bright that they take my mind off on a beautiful tangent.

My friends, this ancient and powerful way of relaxing can help us with mentally winding down and getting a great night's sleep. It is a relaxation and sleep remedy supreme.

If you are someone who loves to be close to nature and gets a sense of rejuvenation and clarity when you do so through camping trips, trekking or whatever it is, then do it as often as you can. This is an incredibly powerful healing activity for your entire being — every single level of it. You will save time, effort and energy, as well as money on doctors' bills, health kicks and associated products, and personal and professional burn-outs. Burn-outs cost us — a lot. If you are an alternative freethinker (and especially if you are a highly successful person who has always done things 'your way'), this philosophy will resonate deeply with you.

Wholistic health means to live well as a regular part of your life. We do not believe that we should wait until disease makes us unwell, and then simply treat the symptoms — often with drugs. Most of us know this approach does not serve the human race well. We know that our bodies, being part of nature, and most definitely intrinsically connected to it, hold the key to our health.

FIT AND CHILLED OUT

You can connect with nature without even being outdoors. You can look out a window onto gardens, or tree tops. Even a tiny window can give you a glimpse of sky and is enough to help settle you into your own private corner of absolute freedom. You can do this for 4 minutes, for 2 hours, or for the length of your favourite album.

It is all nature. Connect in.

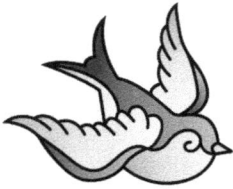

Interview
WITH

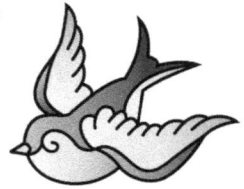

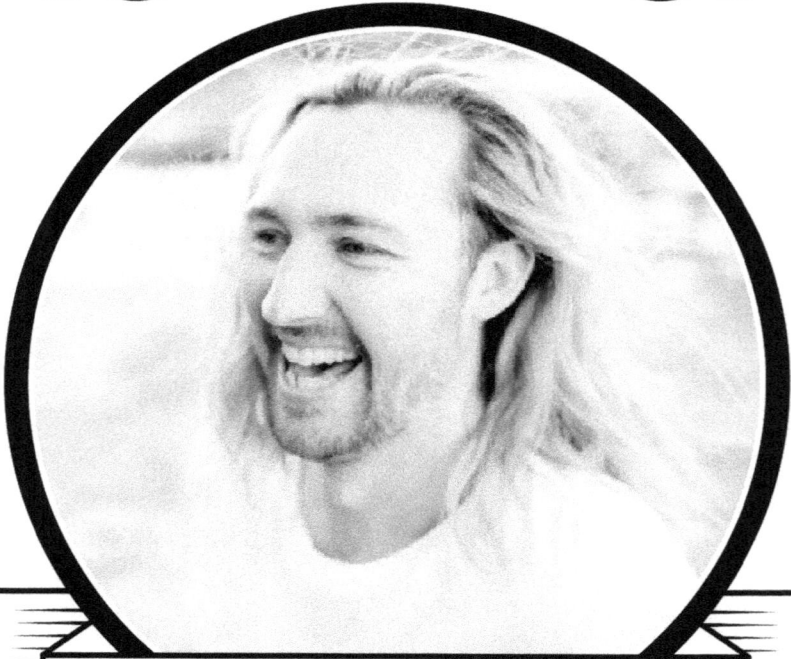

Paul Thompson

✳ Off with your shoes! ✳

FIT AND CHILLED OUT

I really love to support people to tune into the fitness activities and sports that they love most. Through this approach, my members achieve sustainable fitness that they can maintain for the rest of their lives, which inevitably means getting the other well-being results they desire. Paul Thompson is a podiatrist and owner of Corrimal Podiatry. He spoke to me about how to get back into your chosen sport when you haven't played, trained or practiced in quite some time.

- Race: We've been chatting today about mobility and safely returning to your sport, as well as using mobility to enhance safely what you can already do in your sport. So, first of all I wanted to know who's [mobility] for — who could get the most benefits from these kinds of exercises?

- Paul: Mobility exercises are for everyone. Young and old, fit and unfit — but … [surfers], [snowboarders], runners would definitely benefit from the types of exercises [that I teach].

- Race: Okay right, so in terms of being able to get back into the sport that they haven't done in quite some time as well …

- Paul: Yeah, for sure, that's it. [They'll have] less restriction on their joints, less chance of injury, and [they'll be] able to perform better. There won't be as much frustration about why they are not performing like they used to when they were surfing in their 20s. [It] helps you get back to where you were.

- Race: People need [assistance with mobility] in all different areas, don't they? All areas of life. So, could I ask for your take, your unique and expert take, on [what] we need to do [improve our mobility]?

- Paul: Why I do this is to restore natural movement and function, especially to the lower limbs. As a podiatrist, my world is feet, but over the years, I've realised that the whole of each lower limb works as one. So, the more it works as one and without restriction, the better [off] you are.

- Race: [And] the more natural your movement [becomes], the better. This is key, isn't it?

- Paul: Yeah, you stop compensating and you work the way your body was designed to work.

- Race: I've always been fascinated [by how] shoes affect our mobility. Please give me your take on that as well.

- Paul: Paul: Footwear, or traditional footwear, I believe is a curse for most of us. For years, marketing has told us we need more cushioning, more support. From the age of 5, we are thrown into these shoes for school that have anywhere from 10–15 mm of heel height (I know you're a huge fan of high heels, Race … not). Anything over zero is essentially [a] high heel as far as the body or the natural body is concerned. The ongoing effect

67

that has on the rest of our body is insane. It affects the ability of an ankle to … dorsiflex, or bend upwards to its full capacity. Instead, [the ankle] starts blowing off in different positions, so our feet become duck footed to get around the flexion problem, which then causes issues in our hips, our glutes; our pelvis changes direction, we get lower-back pain, all sorts of things. For me, getting barefoot has huge benefits, but of course you need to be safe about it.

- Race: So with barefoot training in particular, [describe] a few of the benefits.

- Paul: From a structural point of view, [barefoot training] helps our body train and move again according to its full range and in a more natural state, so your training is creating a really good behavioural pattern without the shoe doing any work for you. It really gets the feet and the muscles in your feet working hard again.

So, as a podiatrist, I see a lot of problems with shoes. In my opinion, shoes weaken our feet, and that's why I see people and a lot more kids ending up in orthotics, which support the foot even more. We're having to keep supporting the foot rather than taking all that [support] away and actually strengthening the foot. It's like wearing a stiff glove on your hand every day and then wondering why you can't pick up that bit of food. Our feet are the same. They need to move the muscles that are there for a reason. There are a heap of nerves in your feet. There's research around that. [Our feet are] the most nerve-innovated area in our body because we get so much feedback from the ground [through our feet]. [And that feedback] gives our brain so much [information] — if we're on a hard surface, [a] soft [surface], [a] hot [surface], [a] cold [one]. Shoes desensitise everything, shut things off and, to be really negative, can kill our senses.

- Race: Well, I can't wait for you to show me some barefoot exercises!

- Paul: We'll start at the beginning though. You'll do more damage jumping in at the deep end. Mobility, the stuff we're doing today, gets the body moving better, trains the body with that new movement.

Okay, shoes off and we'll do some mobility training!

Watch on Youtube Channel: Star Creatures Wholistic Fitness Retreats

68

FIT AND CHILLED OUT

Ignore me, I'm just having a Zen moment

When a beautiful soul named Naomi (AKA 'Niy Niy') entered my life, we instantly connected and became very close — a soul family. Naomi said numerous witty, memorable and important things to me before she left this planet of ours. Naomi was very proudly of Tasmanian Aboriginal descent, so we held a traditional funeral for her. Our friend Gary was the man who conducted these ceremonies in Sydney. He let us all know, friends and family members, not her say her name out loud after she had returned to her star. I chose to include her name in writing here, so I would like to acknowledge this custom here. We were living in Bundeena, in Sydney's Royal National Park. I was having a giggle at Naomi one day as she was staring into space, happily zoned out. My cheekiness jolted her out of her frozen time, and she cracked up laughing. She said to me, 'I call it having a Zen moment'.

'A Zen moment'. Oh, how many Zen moments I have had. I seem to spontaneously go into Zen moments quite often. When I think about it, I can see that these short spells of stillness are a totally natural (and therefore very common) occurrence for humans. From my experience, I have only ever had them around people whom I feel comfortable with, or if I am alone. I have only seen others have them around me if they are comfortable with me too.

I believe that the Zen moment is to the mind what a yawn is to the lungs: a spontaneous entry into a clear, open space. When the lungs need a large burst of oxygen, our involuntary muscles and impulses make it happen. Similarly, when the mind needs a large burst of clarity and purity, our involuntary brainwaves take us there. It feels so incredibly good to slip back out of it. Always deeply relaxed. Pretty cool, huh? It has simply got to be very good for us.

There is a long word and explanation for it, but we do not need that detail right now. I just wanted to share my sweet memory of Niy Niy with you. May you all be blessed with many a Zen moment!

At times, the human brain needs to slow down and chill for a bit. Relaxing your mind regularly is imperative to maintain good mental health.

Here's a cool 10-minute mental cleanser to try:

- Pick one of these: clouds, trees, stars, waves.
- Let your eyes soften and go out of focus
- Take a deep belly breath
- Watch and simply allow yourself to get drawn in.

It does wonders — try it, and you'll see what I mean.

Chapter 6:
Eat Real Food

I have been interested in food and nutrition for a very long time, from my early martial-arts and dancer days, needing to stay healthy and at a good weight to fuel my body for my highly physical arts.

I became a vegetarian at the age of 22, when I could no longer avoid the reality of what it meant to eat animals. I love animals. I always have. Modern farming is cruel. And gross. Really gross. Not okay. It actually disturbs me, so I can't let myself dwell on it. Instead, I do not eat animals. I do not judge others for their choices, and I no longer answer people's innocent question, 'Why are you a vegetarian?' at the dinner table just as they are about to enjoy their chunk of baby sheep. I just say, 'If you are really interested, that's great, I'll forward you some stuff later'. It is not a good time to be discussing my reasons, as I understand that most people are either in denial (and several of my friends say that they want to stay in denial!) or have a different way of looking at things. I get it. They respect me and my life choices. In my circles, we are a diverse bunch. Our BBQs always start with throwing all the vego sausages and gourmet cruelty-free stuff on the barbie. Once that is done, the meat gets chucked on. Easy-peasy and no drama.

When I was living in Melbourne, I became a volunteer with Friends of the Earth, helping to grow an offshoot collective called 'Real Foods'. There, we met regularly and worked on our daggy little projects. We had to walk through the food co-op to get up to our meeting room. Cool, quirky and inspiring posters and notices covered the walls, advertising everything from farmers markets to rockabilly gigs fundraising for various earth-loving projects. The air always smelled of the earth as I walked through the boxes of organic mangos, cherries, potatoes and onions. This Friends of the Earth group was fabulous. I loved being part of something positive and, having done lots of volunteer work previously, I was more than happy to contribute when work hours allowed. One of the things that I was lucky enough to be involved in was designing and producing a seasonal-foods pocket guide. It showed each season and month of the year and then listed all of the fruits and veggies that were in season. This was a genius idea because there are lots of benefits when you buy what is in season in your agricultural region. I'll list them below.

Professionally, helping people to lose weight, get well, get more energy and get creative when it comes to healthy eating has been one of the absolute favourite parts of my job. I have supported people with different abilities or complex needs to be able to become more independent in their day-to-day lives by feeling good about choosing real food. I have also supported very privileged people who are accustomed to buying everything pre-packaged, which is convenient but expensive. I have been able to teach them that there is nothing convenient about being overweight, undernourished and low in energy. I love cooking, as well as prepping heaps of amazing raw food, including delicious desserts to die for.

I understand that there is a constant stream of advertising selling us substances that barely even resemble real food. I am also aware that we eat for many reasons other than nutrition.

It is a good idea to think about what your reasons are for eating. We all find that there are reasons totally unrelated to nutrition that are absolutely justifiable, such as, 'I love the taste and intensity of curries and chillies', or 'That particular dish reminds me of my grandmother's cooking', or 'It is quick, easy and nutritious as well as yummy'. People can also find reasons that are less positive, such as 'I really crave sugary things when I'm lacking energy', or 'I find that I eat for comfort'. Dudes ... this is okay. Everybody, if they are honest with themselves, has some habits that are not-so-healthy.

At this point in time, during the journey that you're on with me, allowing me to support you by reading my book, you will have already sussed out that I believe in encouraging people and building on positivity. I believe in looking at lots of things from a positive perspective, viewing them as 'adding to' rather than 'taking away from' wherever possible.

Instead of saying, 'I have to stop eating all of the food that I love eating every day... OMG, I'm so scared!', we can use positive language: 'I want to eat lots more of the healthy food that I love eating every day. I'm excited because it is actually easy to do this'. And easy it is. Eat. Real. Food. Eat more real food more often. Eat more. Eat often.

The best advice that I can give you is to keep it simple. The simpler the better. Trust me — it is true. It is actually very easy and is just a matter of giving it time and going with the foods that you love eating. Over time, your taste buds change to appreciate wholesome food. And here's the best bit: you will be able to eat whatever you want. The real magic is that the food you want will change. When you feel like eating your comfort foods or the rich and complicated dishes that you may love having when you go out for dinner, you will do so. The next day, though, you will intuitively start craving fresh, light and tasty vitamin-packed meals again. You become more in tune with your system and your instincts kick in. Some people find that if they are lacking in iron, they will crave iron-rich foods like tabouli and hot-spiced green beans.

Real-food tips

Here are some simple tips to get you eating real food in your daily life:

1. Graze

You won't feel hungry at all when you are constantly grazing. Many people graze these days.
Racing out the door of a morning, it takes under 30 seconds to throw into a bag any combo of real foods to graze on all day — for snacks, lunch, and for the trip home. Take as much as possible so that you have a choice.

For example, I will chuck in 2 large juicy carrots, 2 apples and a mango. I always have my nuts box refilled and ready. Some sweet stuff is always great in the afternoon when I start to fade, and I have found that big juicy Medjool dates are an awesome sweet-tooth tamer. For something more substantial, I will sometimes make a mega-delish burger the night before. I love using a large, tender, baked garlic mushroom as the main act on the burger. I will pull out my stainless-steel lunch box and start munching on roasted almonds the second my tummy starts growling.

Grazing is also amazing for your metabolism. If you eat this way, your metabolism will fly upward through the roof, burning fat at a faster rate. And it will save you time compared to queuing up to grab a salad sandwich, only to find that they have run out of wholegrain and your only option is white bread.

If this becomes a regular practice for you, you will still be able to eat other dishes as takeaway or restaurant dining if you are catching up with friends or celebrating, but you won't be starving by the time you get there. Also, if your regular pattern is to graze on real food all day, at least for half the time, imagine the massive improvement in your health at the end of a couple of months. Better weight, better metabolism, better concentration, and you are directly protecting yourself from future health problems and disease. You can relax, knowing that your nutritional requirements are being met.

2. Buy what's in season

If you buy what's in season locally you will receive a number of benefits:

- Better taste
- Cheaper
- Better quality as no need for freezing or other storage methods
- Better nutritional value because less time is taken from grower to table
- Less likely to be genetically modified as seed saving may be more available to local farming communities

- Reduced environmental impact through less transportation, fuel and energy usage.

3. Never ever say the word 'salad' again

Over the years, I have heard various negative views about salads. A young woman with Down Syndrome whom I was supporting told me flatly, 'I don't like salad'. She hadn't eaten 'salad' for years. I often hear kids (and big kids) say, 'Just the pie and no salad please'. Loving the use of positive language and seeing the transformative effects of it myself, I have stopped using the word salad. A salad simply means a mixture of foods.

The woman who didn't 'like salads' now looks forward to meal-time preparation with me because she gets to choose every ingredient in one of the dishes we make together.

My job in life is to support people to make healthy choices for themselves, and this development was a complete turnaround for the young woman in question. I held up 2 capsicums, a red one and a green one, and asked, 'Which one do you like?'. She chose the red. I then held up an iceberg lettuce and a bunch of kale and asked, 'Which one of these do you prefer?'. She chose the lettuce. Finally, I held up a jar of chickpeas and a bottle of black olives. She wasn't sure, so we opened both and she got to taste them. She loved the chickpeas. This led to the invention of the amazingly exciting dish that she proudly shared with her housemates — not called salad at all, but called 'Red Capsicum, Crunchy Iceberg and Chickpeas'. Which is exactly what it was.

4. Eat clean

I believe that eating clean means selecting wholefoods and organic foods, avoiding genetically modified ingredients, and not adding any nasties like salt, sugar, or saturated fats. There are so many alternatives for these items around that it is very easy to eat clean.

5. Eat more vego food

Even if you could never imagine changing to a vegetarian diet completely, eating more vego food has massive benefits for your health, your weight, for our fluffy and feathered friends, and for the environment.

If you want to eat more vego or vegan stuff for health reasons or for animal ethics, there are lots of alternatives available. Some people buy ethically sound foods when given the option, and every little bit helps. Often, those options are better quality and taste better too.

Some of you may be curious about the nutritional aspects of a vegetarian or vegan diet. Statistics show that vego diets are more nutritionally balanced because we eat a more varied diet. Recent studies have also shown that in some of the richest countries in the world, we have high numbers of people who eat meat regularly but are in fact overweight AND undernourished.

A recent visit to my doctor indicated that my nutritional levels are perfect. Every level of nutrient, vitamin, mineral and essential dietary elements fell within healthy guidelines. Having studied nutrition and knowing that there are several different elements to look at, I thought that something would be a bit low or out of sync. The doctor was impressed with my results, and I had not bothered to mention that I was a vego.

There are hundreds of graphs, tables and lists available to show the nutritional contents of foods. This information indicates which foods are the highest in certain vitamins and minerals. The best part is that as you tune into your intuitive highest self, your Star Creature, you will naturally crave the foods that you need the most. This will happen. It is very easy, my lovely Star Creatures.

6. Prepare a Yummy Healthy Snacking Platter

When I'm really busy writing or working from home, I make up the platter in two minutes the night before and fill it chock-a-block with my favourite goodies. For example, as I write, it's the middle of summer where I live. On my platter are fresh mango and watermelon slices, with a few organic corn crisps topped with sweet tahini. To have later in the day, I added some unsalted tamari roasted peanuts (tamari is a Japanese variation of soy sauce), and 2 large halved carrots, surrounding a simple vegan tomato relish dip that I made yesterday. When I'm having a quick break, or I get my first pangs of hunger between meals, I grab my Yummy Healthy Snacking Platter from the fridge.

7. Eat your largest meal earlier in the day

Going to bed on a full tummy will slow down your system, causing all sorts of problems, including obesity. I usually eat my largest meal for brekky or lunch. For dinner, I will usually whip up something light and protein-filled. I will serve myself up a reasonably sized portion. Dinner time for me is usually that of a 'nanna', at around 4 or 5 pm. That works for me. If I have to meet friends for dinner somewhere later, I will order something small as I won't be hungry. Being a good regular habit, dinner happens this way most of the time for me. If I go through a stage of eating later for a while (say, when I'm super busy or there is a lot of social stuff going on), it doesn't matter. I end up naturally going back into my regular, comfortable routine. Good habits, most of the time, mean flexibility and the ability to have a healthy body and eat in a way that fits in with your lifestyle.

FIT AND CHILLED OUT

Tell me something that I don't already know

In the areas of fitness, health and weight loss, there is an over-saturation of information available, particularly in relation to food — what to eat, what not to eat, when to eat, when not to eat. There are also different ways of looking at food: food combining, calorie counting, high protein, low carb, vitamins and supplements, wholefoods, macrobiotics, raw food — the list is endless. Myriad fad diets go in and out of fashion. Although accessible information is a good thing, the volume of information about our dietary choices (and the mixed messages within that information) can be difficult for the average person to decipher.

We are all different and it is up to each one of us to decide what we put into our bodies (or don't put it in).

Those of us who take an interest in our own health and that of our families have gathered a lot of knowledge along the way. As a fitness professional, I know how much information is out there and how much of it is true and valuable.

My best piece of advice is to draw on what you already know. It is food, not rocket science. You know what works for you and why. You are already aware of the foods and meal habits that make you feel good and the ones that don't. You know that there are certain dishes that you adore that are rich and laden with ingredients that are best enjoyed occasionally and in moderation. Do not feel guilty. Love every second of them and indulge, appreciate, and be in the moment when you eat them. You know that it is best to eat smaller amounts of them. Conversely, you know that there are other foods that are best eaten daily.

Go for it. Eat. Enjoy.

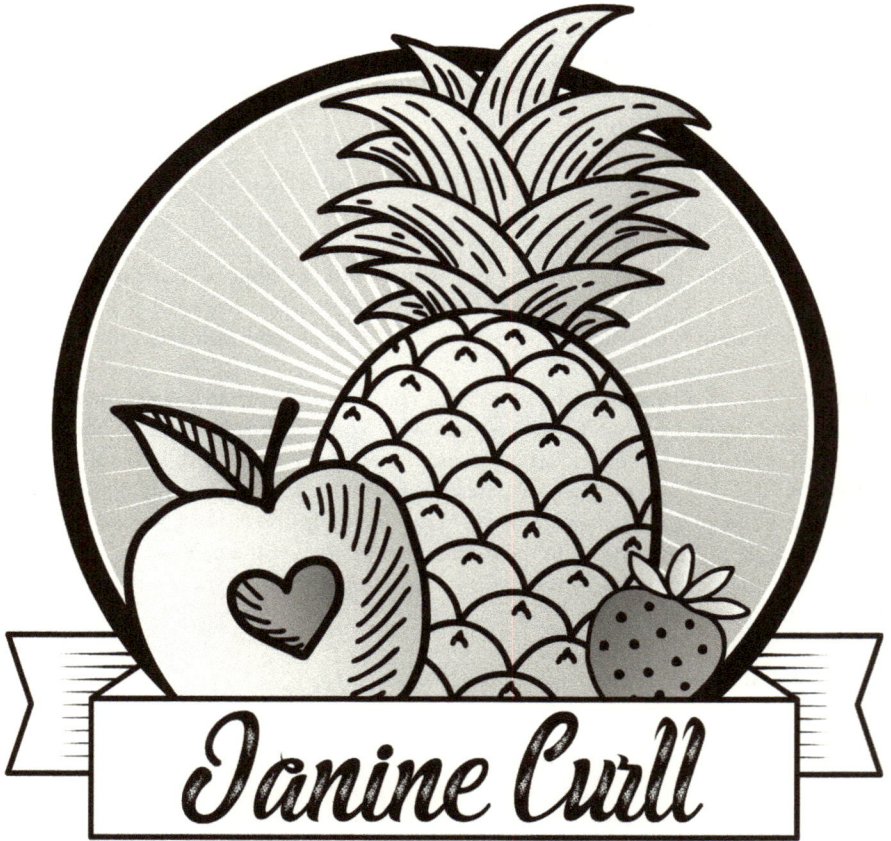

Janine Curll

* Food Fraud *

FIT AND CHILLED OUT

I was so excited when Janine said that she would love to contribute to this book.

Janine Curll BSc LLB MAIFST, PhD Candidate (Monash) in food law and regulation, researches food fraud and the tools to combat it. Janine is the author of 'The Significance of Food Fraud in Australia' (Australian Business Law Review, August 2015). She was a food regulator for the NSW Food Authority, Australia, for 7 years, where she checked mandatory labelling compliance requirements and prosecuted food businesses that intentionally mislabelled foods with prohibited or misleading health claims; false claims of 'organic', 'free-range', 'natural', 'local', 'free from' and country of origin (CoOL) declarations; and false descriptions of meat species and animal welfare attributes.

Food fraud has always been commonplace. In a complex, globalised food-supply system, false descriptions of foods, including the substitution of premium products by diluting, mixing or replacing them with cheaper ingredients, are more common than we think. We cannot conduct our own trace-backs to verify credence claims whenever we purchase food. So, when faced with food-label claims, how can we be confident that we are getting the food that we think we are purchasing? How can we be sure that the foods we buy resonate with our values?

The answer? Think like a detective.

1. Know that premium commodity foods are the most vulnerable to substitution on a global scale, so only purchase from brands you trust. Research reveals that the foods most vulnerable to substitution or dilution are:

Olive oil: Often diluted with every type of inferior oil.

Honey: Found to comprise honey of non-authentic geographic origin, or a mixture of sugar syrup and high-fructose corn syrup instead of authentic bee goodness.

Fish: Researchers have identified high rates of fish species substitution in supply chains around the world, with retailers and restaurants also engaging in substitution (for example, red snapper replaced by cheaper tilapia).

Orange juice: Found mixed with undeclared ratios of other citric juices, such as grapefruit mixed with high-fructose corn syrup, cane sugar hydrolysates, or beet sugar hydrolysates.

Apple juice: Apple juice is often the adulterant in replacement or substitution fraud of other juices. However, apple juice itself has been substituted with high-fructose corn syrup and inverted beet syrup.

> **Coffee:** History of substitution with coffee husks, roasted corn, twigs, roasted barley, roasted soybeans, rye flour, potato flour, roasted date seeds, tamarind seeds, and figs.
>
> **Spices:** Black pepper and saffron – know your supplier or you may score starch, flour, and papaya seeds instead.

2. Buy food in its whole, fresh form. Establish relationships with whomever you purchase your commodities from. Trust your instincts and senses. If it seems too good to be true, it probably is too good to be true. Knowledge of good food combats adulteration.

3. Know that there is no enforceable definition for 'free range'. 'Free-range' claims on foods available in large supermarkets should be considered 'industrialised free range', as the practices are far removed from a consumer's perception of traditional free range. If you must purchase from a leading retailer, look for third-party certification (e.g., organic marks you trust).

4. When looking for food with real-fruit ingredients, look out for the word 'flavoured' in small print, and check the order of ingredients — all ingredients must be declared in the descending order of in-going weight and a percentage must accompany any characterising ingredients — e.g., water, apple (40%), blackcurrant (10%). Don't rely on visual representations of the ingredients; check the back of the label as impressions of fruitiness may be misleading.

5. Therapeutic claims on food, such as 'this product will treat/ cure/ diagnose your ailment/ disease' are prohibited. The presence of these claims is a good indication that the food is snake oil.

6. If nutrition or health claims inspire your purchases, check the Nutrition Information Panel (NIP) and ingredients list to understand the levels of the active claimed ingredients in the food. If there is an antioxidant claim, check the NIP for the listed vitamins. Health claims permitted in the sale of food are based on a systematic review of evidence establishing the food-health relationships. Lab-based in vitro and animal studies do not provide adequate proof of this relationship. Look out for extract declarations and ask yourself whether trace acai extract (for example) will actually deliver any of the claimed nutritional benefits.

7. Food fraud takes place in organic and farmers markets too, so talk to the market holders. Ask questions to understand the nature of their business in an attempt to validate their claims. For example, ask the seller if they can prove the full traceability of a package of meat. If market holders are not forthright and confident in their answers, don't purchase their product.

Chapter 7:

Free Your Mind and the Rest Will Follow

Feed my hungry soul

I was always searching. Searching for an identity. Not just a personal identity but a sense of spiritual self. A clan — my clan. I always felt different from most people. I was certainly highly sensitive to the energy in my immediate environment, more than the average person.

I feel blessed to have had freedom. Freedom to follow my curiosities and passionate drives.

When I was growing up, being such an intense, highly sensitive child and knowing that I could sense the true feelings and intentions of others, I would take pleasure in making them feel 'seen' and loved unconditionally. This tendency was incredible when reciprocated by others who loved me in return. At times though, my attention fed straight into other peoples' egos and I found myself being used, and having roles projected onto me so that other people could play out their own life drama through me. At other times, it felt like I was being consumed as fuel for other peoples' egos. I also felt deeply the fear and resentment that my abilities brought up in some people, particularly those who conducted their lives in less-than-honourable ways. My intuitive gifts, which people close to me have described as a double-edged sword, meant that I was faced with challenging situations growing up. Early on, when these types of people set out to disempower me, I was too young and trusting to defend myself emotionally. Gaslighting and other abusive attempts to control me continued into my adult life. Occasionally, particularly insidious narcissists have been able to get to me when my guard is down (for example, if I am under the weather). Fortunately for me, I was blessed with the warrior's fighting spirit and eventually became so acutely attuned that I can usually detect and deflect these types of attacks. The positive aspects of being able to see into the beautiful souls of people and connect with them most definitely outweigh the bad experiences that may result from this type of gift.

Being the 'pink sheep' of my family, I am the polar opposite to most of my family members in many ways. Being an open communicator, who believes in pulling up the carpet that held all the secret stagnant dust, and that bravery, honesty and kindness lead to healing in relationships, has meant that I have been coldly outcast by some members of my family. This has certainly given me an understanding, on a deep soul level, of how important it is to be included and accepted as 'belonging' (even if you are different) — and how important it is to feel a sense of community.

Without this feeling of belonging, we struggle to provide ourselves with a sense of security and identity. Only the strongest of us get there. I am truly grateful that the universe has provided me with the strength and innate optimism that I possess. I'm also eternally grateful for the truly and unconditionally loving family and friends who continue to appear in my life — the loving kindred spirits and positive souls, brave and like-minded creative beings who have become my soul family. These people mean the world to me, hence the words tattooed on an art piece on my arm, 'Qui con la mia famiglia anima', meaning 'here with my soul family'.

I have so far lived what I consider a very full and exciting life. My circumstances have allowed me to follow my inner voice and the magnetism to explore all things that have inspired me at that particular time. I am genuinely grateful to have had the chance to form as a spirit in an authentic way.

With dance, theatre, music, martial arts and healing as my foundation, I was able to find much creative freedom and identity during the late 1990s and early 2000s, when I explored Sydney's unique, amazing arts and cultural underground. Fronting as a vocalist in live bands, and appearing in some of Australia's best-known performance art theatres, allowed me to work alongside artists who have rocked the very foundations of Sydney's creative arts.

When I was immersing myself in the queer performance art and music underground of Sydney, I became fascinated by this theatrical world. It was in Sydney that it became ultra-cool to have performance art before a live band or other type of gig. Festivals, art gallery openings and nightclubs all started to embrace performance art as the hottest new thing. For me, being a professional dancer and makeup artist for the Mardi Gras, performance art was a cool and exciting new form. I loved the elaborate, over-the-top costumes and makeup looks that I could create. Lots of my friends were fellow artists and we used to say that we were 'in drag' when all glammed-up. Many of us were punky, colourful, pierced and tattooed pixies by day who could easily transform into movie-star-style vixens and pin-up models at night. This is why I still call it drag when I'm getting dressed up. Well, it really is drag. Corporate office drag, conservative cookie-cutter drag, butch-tradesman drag, hipster drag, punk drag. Not only was it a diverse scene of creative and fabulous people, performing all kinds of witty, sexy or moving shows, it was absolutely amazing fitness training. Some of the more elaborate shows needed a lot of rehearsals, and it was a wonderful workout. Creative movement is such a perfect way for me to keep fit because I love it, in all of its forms.

One of my favourite gigs was at the famous Metro Theatre in George Street, Sydney, performing as a support act for DJ Danny Tenaglia. The stage designers built an incredible set, creating a 1920s Berlin red-light district. There were windows from floor to the very high ceiling and we, the dancers, performed intense and high-energy choreography. It was an absolute blast and the funky alternative crowd went absolutely crazy for it.

The art of physical movement and creative freedom has most definitely provided me with some links and keys to knowing how to practice self-care. My wholistic wellbeing has always depended on being able to spread my wings and fly with the seahawks, looking down to pinpoint exactly what is going on in my surroundings as well as in my body.

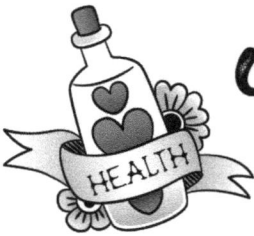

Interview

WITH

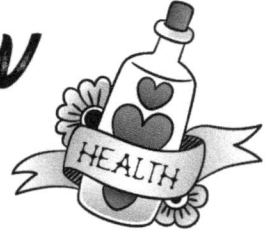

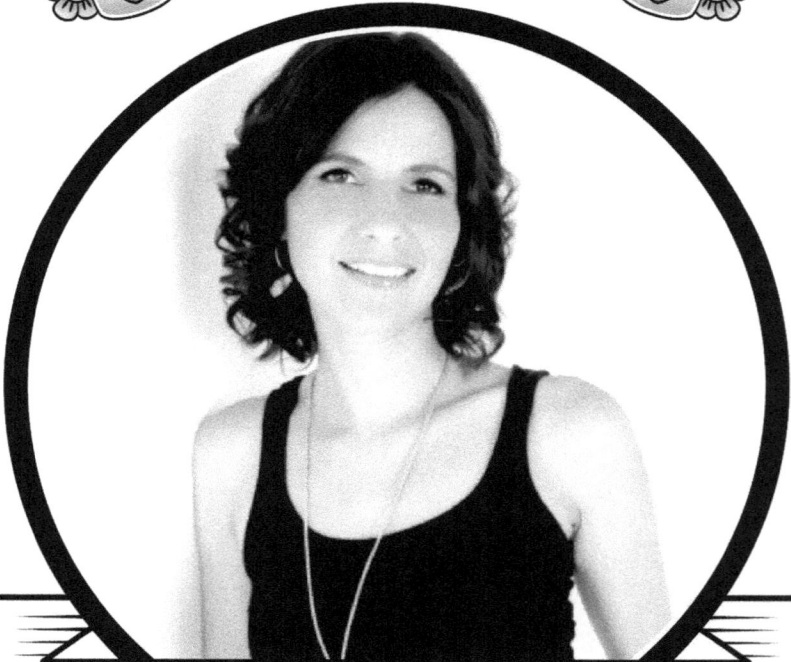

Nikki Gong

✳ Natural Therapies ✳

FIT AND CHILLED OUT

Nikki Gong is qualified in Aboriginal and Torres Strait Islander primary health care, nutrition, fitness, sports and recreation, and community services. She has considerable experience in working with disadvantaged people and has recently developed and delivered some impressive health and wellbeing projects. I've been inspired by Nikki's gentle and caring approach to supporting people on their wellbeing journey — I hope you find inspiration in her words of wisdom too.

Here is the gist of my chat with Nikki about the value of natural therapies:

- Race: Why do you believe in natural therapies?

- Nikki: I believe in natural therapies because of the results [they deliver]. Something I really noticed when I started learning about natural therapies is that the body's got this amazing ability to heal itself, if it's given the right tools. That [discovery] was huge for me — with natural therapies, the body is able to heal itself [if it's] given the right things to heal with; it's the body's natural state to be able to heal itself. That's why I so strongly believe in [natural therapies]. People get results [from natural therapies] because the body is naturally supposed to [heal].

- Race: What's the best approach to [utilising] natural therapies alongside medical intervention?

- Nikki: Yes, this is a good [point]. So, for me, I've found that natural therapies are great at prevention — preventing disease and preventing illness. Natural therapies are a great way to treat an illness, [while] the medical side of things [does] really well at diagnosing [disease]. So, in an ideal world, it would be perfect for [natural therapies and medical intervention] to work together. I think medicine does have a really important role in emergency care and it definitely has its place. There is a real need for medicine and Western medicine — operations and emergency care, broken bones, and those kinds of things. I think the best thing would be complementary medicine, where [the two modalities] are working together.

- Race: People will be really interested in that too. There's often that cross-section, people get a bit overwhelmed about doing the right thing and going into the direction that everyone else feels confident in.

- Nikki: That's right. The best thing about complementary medicine is [to] be educated and informed about options. There are different ways of treating things and it's really important that people know what their options are.

- Race: What are the main things you love about natural therapies?

- Nikki: I love [natural therapies] because they're wholistic. Natural therapies incorporate all different types of health, like physical health, emotional health, mental health, spiritual health. [All aspects of health are] really important.

Wholistic heart and soul – volunteering

Over the last 12 months, while designing the perfect support plan for my Star Creatures, it went without saying that volunteering would be central to the philosophy. As part of our International Star Creatures Wholistic Fitness Retreats, we give guests the option of taking a road trip to a not-for-profit organisation, to do skills sharing or to lend a hand. I have called this the 'Wholistic Heart and Soul Project'.

At the moment, I am associated with a Balinese orphanage run by volunteers. As part of their fitness practices during their stay, our retreat guests will have learned a series of beautiful martial-arts-based movements (kata), which they can then teach to the children in the orphanage. Children love to learn new things, and for our guests to be able to share these skills is fantastic. As a group, we may also do a shopping run for the centre, or help with anything else that the staff need.

In my retreats and in the work that I do with my members, I place a strong emphasis on simple balance. I believe that maintaining a healthy spiritual self is every bit as important as physical health because it is all connected. Thus, I am a strong believer in supporting those in need through sharing our energy.

Whilst financial assistance and donations are essential to enable not-for-profit groups and organisations to exist and to function, I believe that it is volunteers who become the backbone of these important causes.

Volunteering has a magical element — it brings human beings together to work for a common purpose, and that is always a positive thing.

Throughout my life, I have volunteered with many not-for-profit organisations, usually whilst working full time. I started volunteering when I was in my early 20s. My favourite time of year to volunteer is at Christmas because there is a different vibe in the air amongst the tribe of volunteers. It is a gathering of souls for a higher purpose, so you connect deeply. I have met some unbelievable people whilst volunteering. It is ironic that often, the busiest people are the ones who volunteer. Doers get more done.

Do you really live where you live?

Like a lot of other important things in life, weighing up the pros and cons of our living location is something that is absolutely worth considering. Bear in mind that I am speaking in terms of the most important aspects of your life here: your health, fitness and wellbeing. We have covered all the reasons why this perspective is important, and we need to keep this in the forefront of our minds. A healthy, fit, chilled-out and happy you is going to be a better partner, parent, entrepreneur, artist, kick-ass mover and shaker, and world changer. Prioritising your wellbeing is also a great way to keep big decisions in perspective.

Parents have a particularly hard time getting their heads around this theme of prioritising their own health and wellbeing above anything else. I like to think of the aeroplane safety instructions analogy. We are always told to secure our own oxygen mask before attending to others, including our children. I never understood that until I was older, but now I realise that we are not much help to anyone else if we cannot breathe. That principle holds in our day-to-day lives too.

Prioritising our wellbeing is a great opportunity to put some real time and thought into the question, 'Do I really live where I live?'.

For me, I know that, wherever possible, it is best for me to live in a quiet place that is near the ocean. Nature is important for me. Wellbeing needs to be my top priority. Everything else must be placed further down the list. The pure waters of life must flow off the healthy solid rock of my being.

Also, high up on the priority list is that I need to be around chilled-out people, and others who do not subscribe to mainstream stuff and relate more to alternative cultures. Occasionally, I need to go to reggae and rock gigs and to see live alternative performances that move me. I need to sometimes be in the company of fun, freethinking people that I can relate to and who 'get me', and I enjoy having long, deep and meaningful conversations with other spiritual and heart-centred people.

Recently, whilst travelling home from a spontaneous camping trip with a friend, the subject of where she lived came up in conversation. Being a naturally gifted psychic who is extremely talented in the medium of palmistry, she told me she needed a lot of time alone, in a very peaceful environment, in order to restore her energy. She loves socialising; however, many of our friends live in the city, so it has become less of a priority. But, having chosen a home that is around a one-hour drive from town, she is still able to socialise when she wishes to do so.

This conversation with my friend is a perfect example of someone who has found the perfect place to live in order to keep everything in their life in balance.

Obviously, there are a huge number of things to consider when choosing where to live, including house prices or rental costs, the cost of living, distances to work and schools, and so on.

With your health, fitness and wellbeing as your main focus, make a list of questions, or pros and cons, regarding where you live. Here are some suggestions:

- How do I feel about my general surroundings?
- How easily can I access my activities for fun fitness?
- How easily can I nurture myself on a wellbeing level?
- What are my top fitness and wellbeing priorities and how easily can I achieve these?
- What are the other life priorities that need to link in with these?

You can also try listing the general pros and cons of where you're living now, and the pros and cons of moving to where you would love to be.

The objective of the exercise is to take a look at your current priorities and, from there, examine your options. More options tend to surface when you examine these questions on a deeper level.

Live and let live, love and let love

To live is to thrive, to sparkle and shine. To feel free. To be fit and strong. To be supported by others to be all that you can be. To live and love life. To be grateful to be alive. To love the people who are important to you by giving them the freedom and dignity to live their own lives the way that they want to. To look at the people that you love and to smile, knowing that they are on their own soul journey, one that you are connected to in some way. To feel balanced within yourself, most of the time.

Listen more often to the people you love. Hear their words in your heart more often. Wish peaceful and personal wellbeing on the people you love. Ask to be listened to. Ask for help. Communicate from your place of deep truth. Be calm and brave, as the truth will always shift energy from heavy to light. Be kind. Celebrate all of our differences as well as our similarities.

Love life, love your own evolution, and love the beautiful souls that we get to share our time here with. Let yourself off the hook when weighed down by what someone else is doing. We are separate beings — separate, but connected by love.

Synchronicity

Many of us believe that coincidences and déjà vu do not happen by chance.

Books and teachings from around the world have drawn the same conclusion. I remember reading a book called the Celestine Prophecy in the early 1990s, which aligned deeply to my innate sense of faith and spirituality. Other books awakened my interest in metaphysics, including The Holographic Universe. My personal experiences in the areas of interdimensional communications and out-of-body experiences were backed up by what I already knew to be true. As a child and throughout my life, my views on this topic have been confirmed through my experiences. I am absolutely convinced that there is more to our earthly dimension than meets the eye. The Secret was another book popular in the early 2000s, and although I was already familiar with and had incorporated things like manifestations and approaches such as 'like attracts like' into my life, I still saw value in reading it. I found it interesting that such a book was able to speak not only to the converted like myself but also to the mainstream masses. The book resonated with a lot of beautiful evolved souls who may have had strong talents and gifts but who were unable to explain some of their synchronistic experiences to date. This book awakened many readers to the truth of the beauty, simplicity and easy accessibility of abundance and 'dreaming'.

Some of you have been lucky enough to be blessed with cultural knowledge in these areas, or family openness about the magic of the universe. Or you will have had access to extensive information sources about these themes, and are highly educated on them.

Synchronicity is love. Synchronicity is flow and the acceptance that movement and shifts happen in due time. Synchronicity is seeing signs — signs that show us when we are on the right track and when we need to retrace our steps back to the clearly-lit path. Synchronicity is when we think about someone, only to bump into that person in an unlikely place. Synchronicity is recognising that, although we have missed the bus, we still arrive at work at the perfect time to experience the day that is meant to be.

It is funny, mysterious and magical how often the signs and messages we receive are so extremely random, showing up as things that could be only a chance in a million. I believe that signs like these enable us to really 'get it'. Signs make us aware that something is truly significant, with a deep meaning behind it. My mates and I smile knowingly when things are on the right track — a feeling we have affectionately named 'synchro'.

Chapter 8:

Magic Potions
(Get Fit and Chilled_Out by Having Fun)

From diluted spirit to Star Creature

In the process of reading this book, many of you may have identified that you have indeed been suffering from a diluted spirit. Of course, this condition is very serious — it prevents people from living a full life. Although this may sound extreme, no doubt you can see now that it is true. If you haven't yet found a sustainable way of being fit, healthy and relaxed, you will find that you continue to go around and around on the rollercoaster of fads and phases, resulting in fluctuations in your moods, weight, and wellbeing. Clearly, this has flow-on effects throughout your whole life, including the level of success you are able to achieve personally and professionally. It reduces your ability to reach the highest possible levels of accomplishment in the areas of your life that matter most to you.

Having travelled this far along the journey of this book with me, you will have pieced together that what I do, as a fitness professional and intuitive support person, is take my members, retreat guests (and now you as my reader) through my methodology in a way that will make perfect fitness and optimum wellbeing genuinely sustainable for you.

When we are starting off in a place of diluted spirit, knowing that our true spirit is being blocked from shining through, we can start to go through the basic processes of my methodology in order to reach the highest possible version of yourself. Your Star Creature is the fittest, happiest, most chilled-out, most balanced, most compassionate, most successful, most progressive and evolved human being that you can be.

As you can see from this methodology, becoming a Star Creature is not stressful. It is not expensive or difficult. It is not even uncomfortable. In fact, it is easy. It is effortless. It is an amazing, wondrous journey into identifying the unique universe that is you. Growing, building and expanding … you. Glowing you. Shining you. The you that makes a mark on the world and that achieves precisely what you are on this earth to do: your soul's calling. It is impossible to achieve this while you are functioning in a stagnant state of diluted spirit. But, once you are powered in your Star Creature mode, magic happens.

When working closely with my members, my team and I are able to tap deeply into achieving this quickly and accurately. My inspiring long-term members, whom I have had the privilege of getting to know very well, have shown me that they are able to click directly into highly effective sustainability in their fitness and wellbeing practices through ongoing support, reconnecting with like-minded people and taking the time to remember all the important self-work that they have done to get them to this level of awesomeness.

To the high fliers in successful alternative companies who impact the planet on a daily basis, to the creative freethinkers who have climbed to the top of all sorts of ladders and broken patterns and stereotypes in the process, to the people who clear their own path through the thick jungle for the like-minded ones to follow, I have been blessed to have worked with you. At the same time, I feel blessed to have had the opportunity to become an author and to share my simple but hugely powerful framework with you.

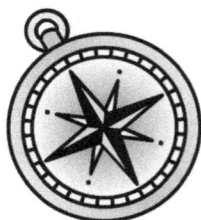

Interview
WITH

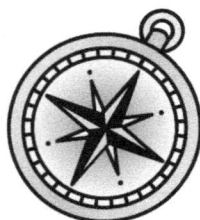

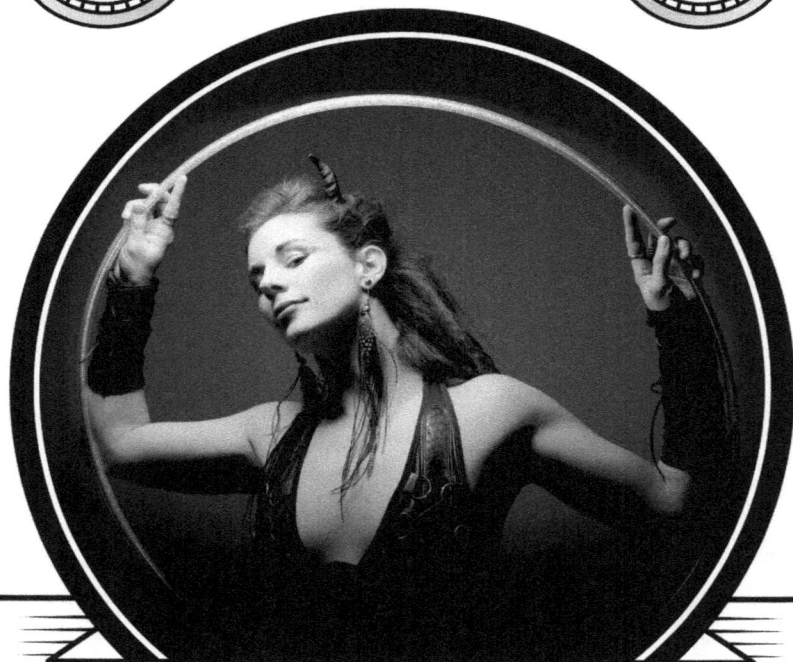

Bahz Robinson
✳ Hula Hooper ✳

FIT AND CHILLED OUT

Let me introduce you to Babz Robinson, who is a hoop art extraordinaire from Canada and a YouTube star who has run workshops in Australia. She's someone who has really nailed the idea of making exercise fun! I had the opportunity to speak with Babz on her recent visit to Australia.

- Race: First thing I wanted to talk about was that, you know, you're an amazing high flyer in your art and that comes across in everything you do. I'd really love to hear about how cool the hooping community is and why it's so aligned with … alternative cultures.

- Babz: I think one of the reasons why [hooping is] still in the alternative cultures is that a lot of the exposure [of the art] has come from festivals and music events, where a lot of people see hula hooping as an alternative lifestyle event. But hula hooping is so awesome because it's very inclusive. You don't have to fit into a certain mould to be a hula hooper, you know. You don't have to dress a certain way or fit into something. It's also a really good creative outlet. With a lot of exercises or sports, there's a right way to do it, and with hula hooping there is no right way and there's no wrong way. You can be yourself and create your own movement.

- Race: Absolutely, and that comes through in the different styles [of hooping] that you guys [practice]. It's one of the things I love about [hooping].

- Babz: [Hooping is] sort of, I guess, quite dance-based, so if you like dancing it's like having a dance partner, if you will.

- Race: Right, okay, I'm also really keen to know what kind of special gifts you bring as a teacher and coach as well. I really love sort of helping people tune into what they do in their life that makes them feel unique, so I'd love to hear about what you've been put on this planet to do individually, that you can give to your students, that is your special gift to them.

- Babz: I have been putting out You-Tube tutorials for quite some time, and that's where I've found my place in the [hooping] community — as a teacher. As I mentioned, hooping can be really creative, and I've created my own move sand [put] that out and [shared it] with the community. And everybody in the community is welcome to do that as well. It's not like only certain people can come out with things. But through my tutorials, I really put my own flavour into my tutorial, and we don't really — most tutors don't take themselves too seriously or take hula hooping too seriously. It is a plastic circle and it is, like, a child's toy.

- Race (laughing): [A] beautiful plastic circle, sparkly.

- Babz: [Hooping is] about play and when I teach workshops and classes I really like to remind everybody that we're just here to have a good time and play. I like to inspire people through my own expression.

- Race: And that you do, and people know when they watch your tutorials

91

that they're also learning stuff that's a world first, which must be really exciting for your students. Obviously, you love what you're doing. The minute you start [hooping], your face just lights up and you look beautiful and in your element. What I'd like you to share with everybody is your opinion on physical fitness, specifically the fitness benefits, that people get from hula hooping across the board.

- Babz: I would say coordination. I've heard from a lot of people where [hooping has] increased their hand-eye coordination dramatically. Whenever somebody throws something at me now it's like, 'Nice catch'. And just mobility in your joints, 'cause you're moving all kinds of different ways, also increasing body awareness — lots of those, you know, weird, hard-to-tone muscles.

- Race: Absolutely.

- Babz: Anytime you've got a hoop in your hand, you are using those muscles. As well, [hooping is] quite [a] full body [activity], 'cause you're not just hooping on your body, you're hooping on your chest, or on your shoulders or elbows, depending on what you want to do. If you're working on something specific like muscle groups, you can find specific hoop movements that target those as well, so cardio, weight loss, coordination — also the mind-body [connection] — yeah, it's pretty hard to have a bad time [hooping]! Give anybody a hula hoop and as soon as they start, you watch this smile spread across their face. It's just fantastic. You just feel really good.

- Race: Thank you, it's been awesome interviewing you.

Watch on Youtube Channel: Star Creatures Wholistic Fitness Retreats

FIT AND CHILLED OUT

If it doesn't exist, create it

Recently, a fabulous friend of mine told me that she had rediscovered some of her favourite relaxation styles, and that she had started to do lots of hiking for exercise while away camping. As a professional dancer, she had been mega fit, and she wanted to get that body and vibe back into her being. All of the dance classes she had looked into, however, didn't sit right with her, and she realised that she needed a class for ex-dancers, which (as far as she knew) did not exist.

Make it exist, I said. There are numerous platforms for group-gathering these days, so it is very easy to bring together like-minded people. A few years ago, when I wanted to find other peeps who loved bushwalking as much as I do, I posted a free LGBTQI community hiking group. In the process, I not only met new friends but was able to provide a healthy option for people to connect socially.

In the areas of wellbeing, I have started my own support groups as well as meetup groups for fellow empaths, and other groups that had not existed previously. The magic of you can grow in many different ways, my beautiful stars — believe me.

Chapter 9:

Manifesto

Our planet Earth, and its air, water, fire, soil and spirit, lives in energy, breathes through the trees and loves through the creativity and spontaneity of life. We are all truly blessed to be here, and we are all truly loved. Loved by the very life force that gave us the original magical twinkle that created our life.

Every human being on this beautiful, gigantic planet of ours carries the superpowers of physical, mental, emotional and spiritual layers of being. Each one of us is a complete perfect universe intact. Leave a legacy. Write a manifesto. Share it with your world.

Here is mine. I call it my **Manifesto for a Peaceful Life:**

- Identify my true heart's desires throughout my life. Use my natural fire, my determination and my ambition to do my best action to enable these desires to manifest.

- When I think of a creative way to go about attaining these desires, do so in a steady, balanced fashion.

- During the moments that I am not directly working on these things, let them go. If they are meant to be, my positive action will set the energy spinning in motion, and it will have the best possible chance of being swirled up by the universal powers in order for these things to come into being.

- In my day-to-day life, use my mindfulness practice to stay in the moment. Be truly 'present' while working, walking, shopping or exercising. Guide myself back to my Zen. Be mindful to appreciate the gift of beauty in random moments.

- Sparkle and shine every day in my life, while alone as well as out in the world as my life is happening right now. There is nothing to wait for. Share with others my most heart-centred and beautiful self and see the highest Star Creature in others.

- Appreciate my privileges in life. In my free time, when I have the luxury of

- doing whatever my heart desires, connect and check in. Ask myself what I need to do right now. Plan to do these beautiful things for fun and to live the fullest life possible. Identify my basic grounding needs, including my relationships and connection to all things that make me feel safe, secure and held.

- Honour the fact that this amazing planet and my life itself offer freedom to do an uncountable number of positive and soulful things. I have choices. I can go hiking or take a walk on a beach. I can go to a dance class, spend some time with friends, make some art, or go out dancing until dawn.

- Appreciate every moment of free time as the golden times and bliss in life. Life changes. The amount of free time varies throughout life. Sometimes important duties call. Sometimes free time is abundant. Fully appreciate and honour my gift of freedom.

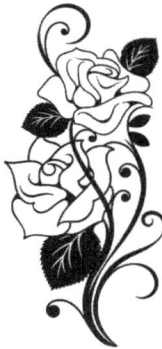

I would like to send out a big, etheric, warm thank you to everyone who contributed to the first edition of this book. I hope you all agree that it was worth the long wait!

Although I wrote this book in 2015, my life changed dramatically in the time period that followed. I finally received the divine green light to begin living the dreams I had manifested for so long. Not for the first time in my life, I left my birthplace of Sydney, Australia, to follow the siren song of another destination.

This time, that place was tropical Far North Queensland. It was here, in this ancient, wild paradise, that I began raising twin toddlers who needed a second chance at life. Since then, my incredible and adored 'bubba girls', Xena and Ella, have become the two most important people in my world. Their names conjure images of warrior princesses, and my girls most certainly have fighting and regal spirits. The last few years have been the most important time in my twins' lives. With this in mind, one hundred percent of my time, resources and loving energy needed to be showered on these wonderful little people. It has been the greatest honour of my life to watch them thrive.

This year, in 2019, my girls have confidently settled into their first year of school life. As a result, I have now had a little free time to birth my book. I believe in divine timing, always.

In order to really get the most out of this book, my recommendation is to return to my interviews with other like-minded souls for inspiration from time to time. As part of your commitment to welcoming my framework into your day-to-day life, it is also important to revisit the book's methodology section at regular intervals. It is in that section of the book, in particular, that you can connect and re-connect with my true intention and find the authentic power of achieving inevitable, lifelong wholistic fitness.

Love fully, start each day with a grateful heart, and enjoy life to the max.

Race

www.ingramcontent.com/pod-product-compliance
Lightning Source LLC
Chambersburg PA
CBHW031217270326
41931CB00006B/598